WHEEL EXCITEMENT

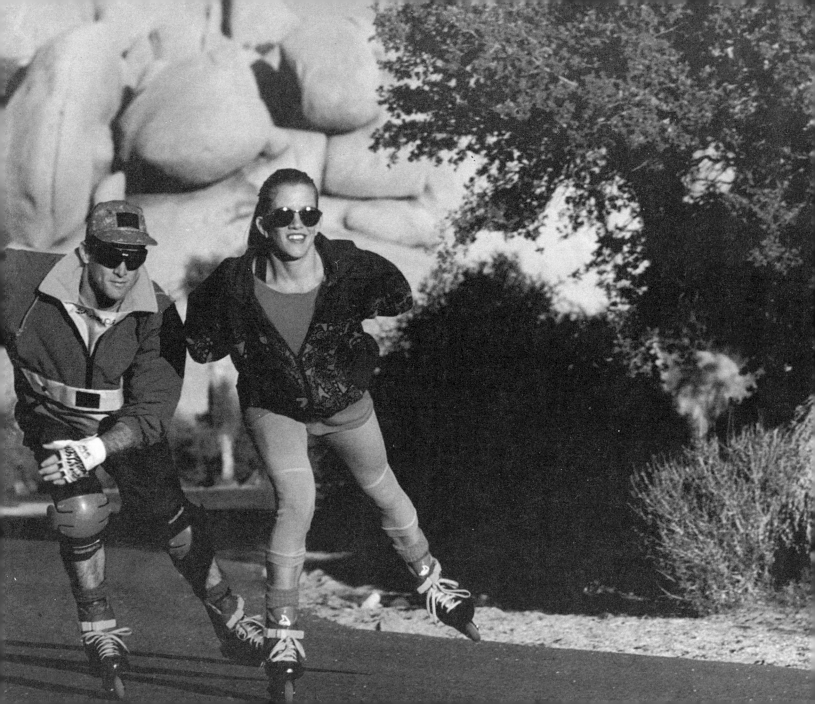

BY NEIL FEINEMAN
WITH TEAM ROLLERBLADE®

WHEEL EXCITEMENT

THE OFFICIAL ROLLERBLADE® GUIDE TO IN-LINE SKATING

PRODUCED BY ALISON BROWN CERIER BOOK DEVELOPMENT

HEARST BOOKS / NEW YORK

Library of Congress Cataloging-in-Publication Data
Feineman, Neil.
Wheel excitement: the official Rollerblade® guide to in-line skating / by Neil Feineman with Team Rollerblade®.
        p.   cm.
"Produced by Alison Brown Cerier Book Development."
ISBN 0-688-10814-8
        1. Roller-skating.   I. Title.
GV859.F45 1991
796.2'1—dc20

Photographer Credits
All photographs by Bruce Benedict except: Greg Benson, page 108; Jill Greer, page 141; Ken Greer, pages 6, 15, 16; Rick A. Kolodziej, pages 124, 129, 130, 132 (top); John Lehn, pages 2, 14, 28, 46, 68, 83, 94, 139; Scott Markewitz, page 51; Rick Sferra, page 27.

Printed in the United States of America
First Edition
1 2 3 4 5 6 7 8 9 10
BOOK DESIGN BY BINNS & LUBIN / BETTY BINNS

ACKNOWLEDGMENTS

This book could not have happened without the generous assistance of many people. Many thanks to Doug Boyce, Bruce Jackson and Chris Edwards for their help with the extreme skating chapter; Karen Edwards, Jonathan Seutter and Dave Cooper for the race chapter; Dean Hart for the gear chapter; Douglas Brooks and Dr. Carl Foster for the workouts; John Sundet, Mary Horwath, Kae Peterson and the rest of the Rollerblade gang for their support; Jill Schultz and Chris Morris for going well beyond the line of duty; and Lisa Boelter of *Beach Culture* for her eyes and computer expertise.

Thanks also to Bruce Benedict for his inspired how-to photographs and to Anne Entwistle for making the photo shoot happen. Special thanks to Joe Janasz and Alison Brown Cerier, because the book just wouldn't have gotten done without them.

And thanks to all the in-line skaters across the country who provided information for this book.

CONTENTS

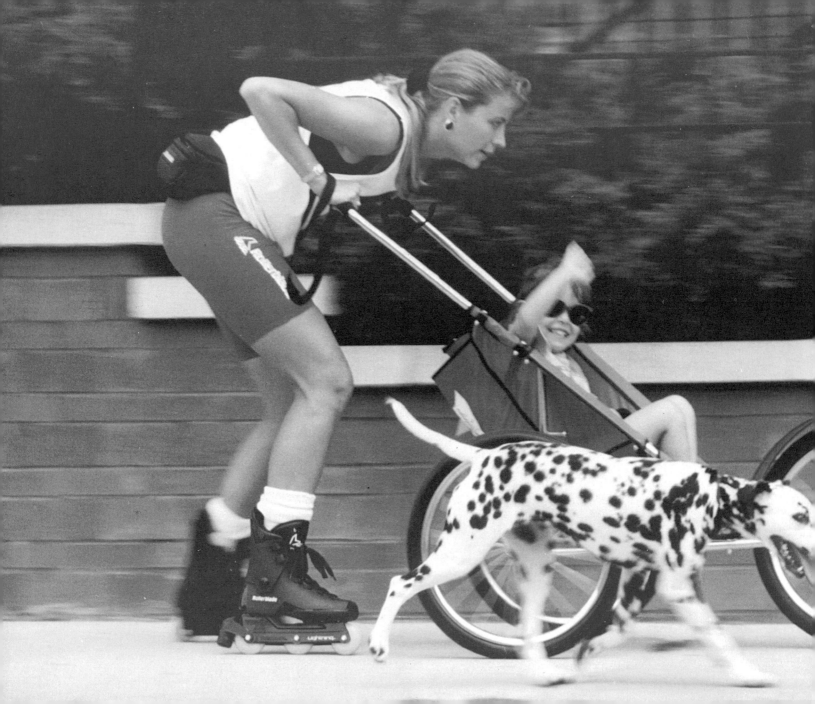

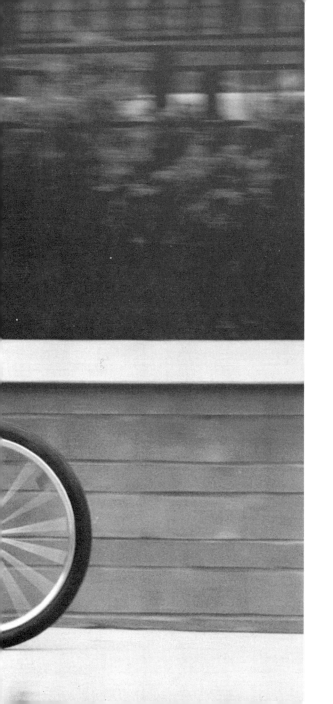

IN-LINE, IN-LIFE

1

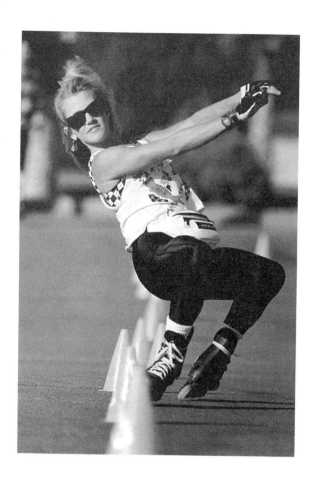

Suddenly in-line skates are everywhere. From MTV to *Fortune* magazine. From Los Angeles to New York and points in between. From the streets to the bike paths to the hockey rinks, in-line skates have captured the imagination of the media, the athletic community and now the country.

An exaggeration? Not when the numbers of in-line skaters swelled from a mere twenty thousand in 1984 to over one million in 1990. Or when retail sales exploded from a previous high of $20 million in 1989 to an estimated $150 million in 1990.

Even more encouraging are the diversity of the people using the skates and the ways they are using them. All ages, from six to over sixty, are working out, racing, dancing, playing rollerhockey or just plain having a good time on them. In the process, they are laying the foundation of what is certain to become a major sport.

No matter how differently they use the skates, everyone from the most radical ramp skaters to the ultramarathoners to the Sunday-afternoon skaters has two things in common. First, everyone is having fun. Second, each is burning calories and getting fit. In fact, an important new study by Dr. Carl Foster, coordinator of sports medicine and sports science for the United States Speed

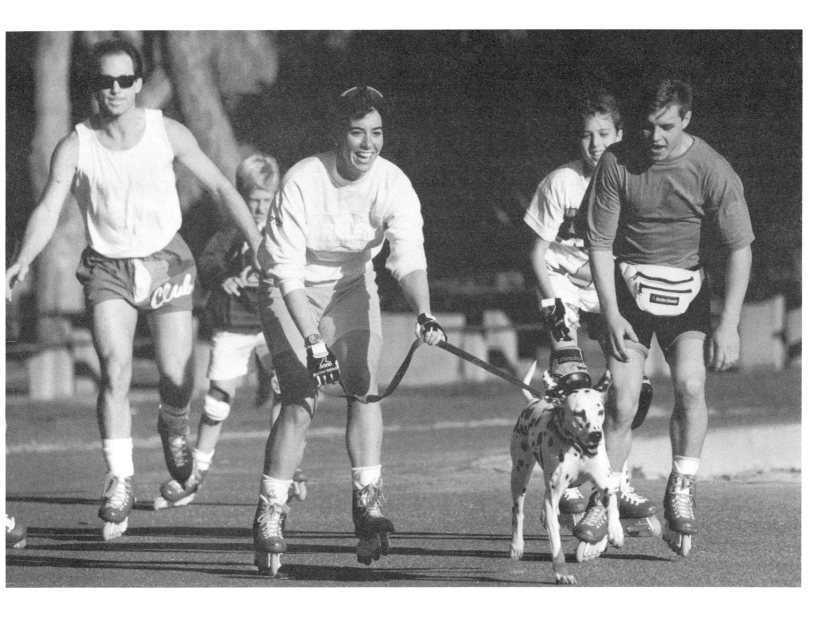

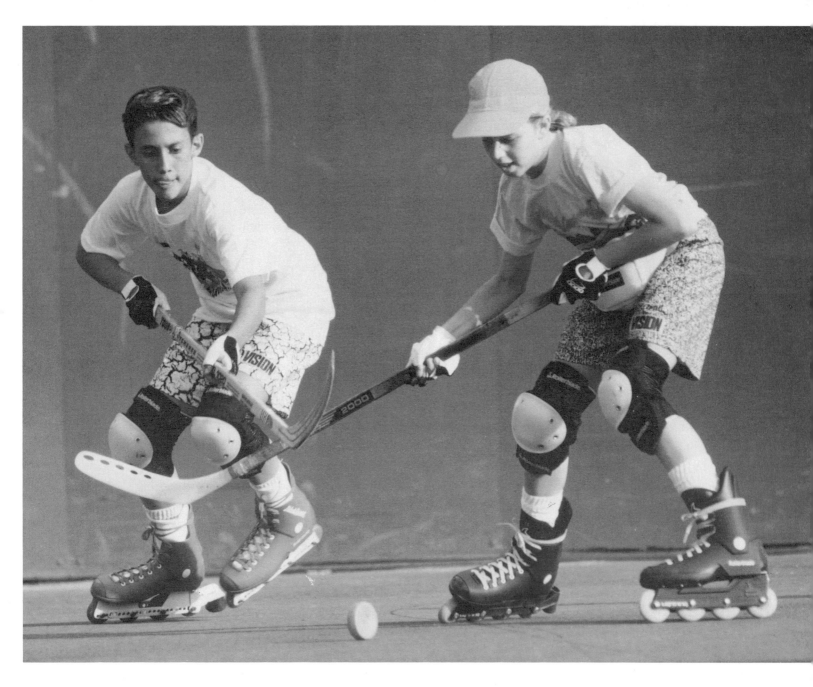

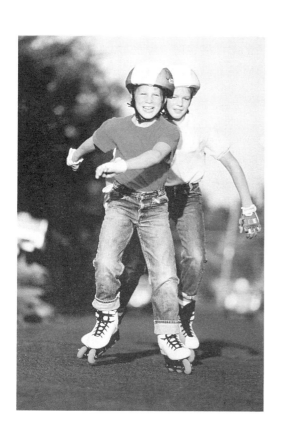

Skating Team, has now conclusively proved that in-line skating is a tremendously effective form of exercise.

His study showed that a person who skates recreationally for thirty minutes burns an average of 285 calories. A proficient skater, moreover, can burn about 450 calories in the same thirty minutes, making the aerobic workout even more effective than a straight running or cycling workout.

Because of the glide, moreover, in-line skating is a low-impact activity. There is none of the pounding of running, and therefore there are none of the associated overuse injuries, such as shin splints and knee problems.

Yet, surprisingly, in-line skating uses and develops more muscles of the legs, hips and thighs than running or cycling. If you want to tone your muscles—and who doesn't?—at the same time you are burning calories and fat, in-line skating is actually a better workout than either running or cycling.

For these reasons and others, in-line skating is an excellent way to cross train. Runners and aerobic dancers can appreciate the relief from the impact of their sport; cyclists can get off the saddle but keep their lower-body strength; swimmers can round out their upper-body workout by developing the lower body. In addition to building strength and conditioning, winter athletes—hockey players, Alpine or Nordic skiers or ice skaters—can work on specific skills such as poling, edging and striding.

In-line skates may sound too good to be true, but after all, the idea has been almost three hundred years in the making. The first skate, an in-line model, was developed in the early 1700s by a progressive Dutchman who tried to simulate ice skating in the

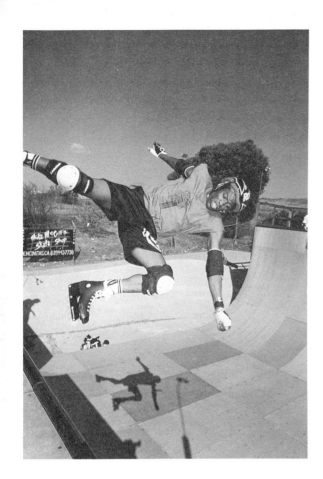

summer by nailing wooden spools to strips of wood and attaching them to his shoes.

The next in-line skate appeared about fifty years later, when Joseph Merlin, an instrument maker in London, decided to dazzle a masquerade party by skating in on metal-wheeled boots while playing a violin. The entrance was made even splashier when he realized he had forgotten to learn how to steer or stop, giving new meaning to the phrase "crashing a party."

The concept remained more or less dormant for the next 220 or so years. Then, in the early 1980s, a group of Minneapolis hockey enthusiasts came up with the idea of using a skate with a single row of wheels in off-season training.

The primitive skates worked. Friends and friends of friends didn't want to miss out, and got their own. Before long, there was a burgeoning local market for the skates. From such humble beginnings, Rollerblade, Inc. and the in-line skate were born.

Although word of mouth fueled increasing demand, until about 1985 everyone thought of the skate as an off-season, hockey-related product. Then, in 1986, skiers discovered them. A year later, it was ever-alert Southern California's turn. Rollerblade, Inc. realized the skates weren't being used just for cross training, but because they were fun in and of themselves.

After that came the explosion. The media couldn't get enough of the skates. They jumped on the bandwagon and stayed on.

Unlike other "flavor-of-the-month" fads, in-line skating has grown bigger and better each year. The numbers continue to double annually. Even more importantly, the skaters are beginning to band together in subcultures, organize informal competitions and

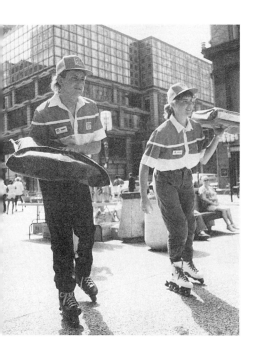

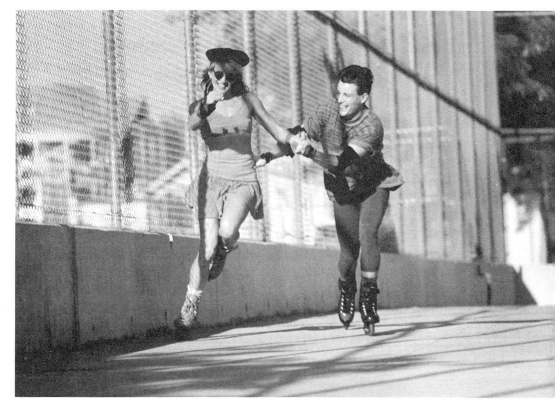

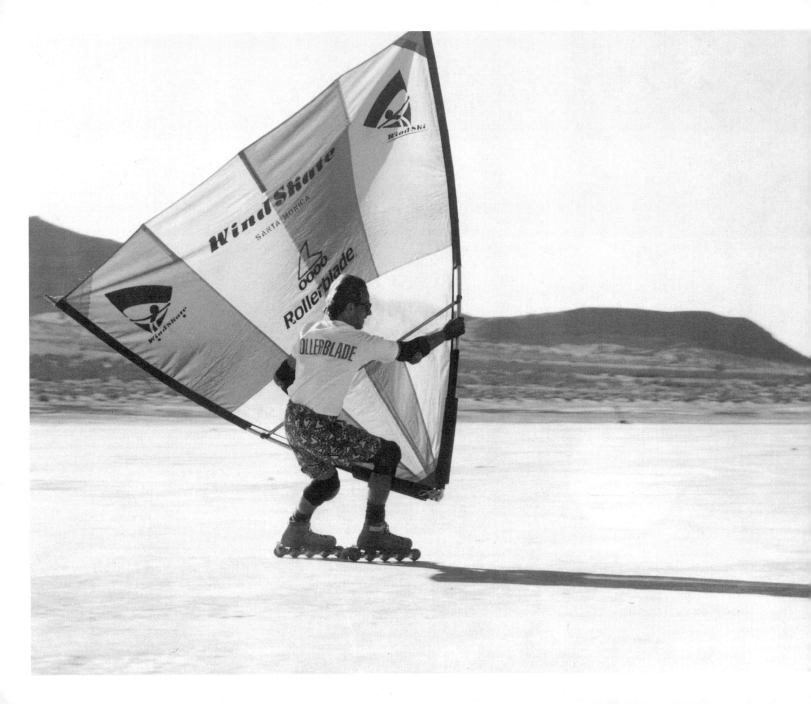

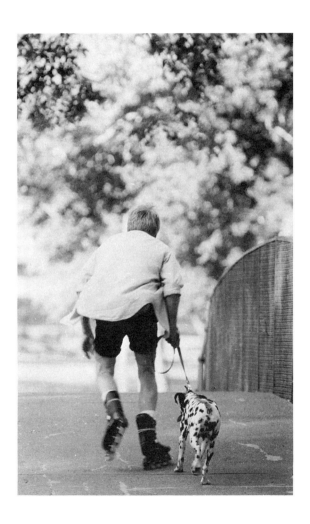

make the first steps toward turning the activity into a full-fledged sport.

These efforts became much easier in 1990, when Rollerblade, Inc. organized RISA™, the Rollerblade In-Line Skate Association™. It is an industry-wide organization dedicated to creating and promoting standards, rules and guidelines for all facets of in-line skating, including safety, competitions and trails. For the first time, the sport has a governing body that is interested in its long-term, sensible growth.

This book will lead you through the basic skills and show you how to become fit through the Rollerblade 30-Minute Workout™. Then it will introduce you to the directions your skating can take, from races to cross training to rollerhockey to stunts and artistic moves.

If something sounds like fun, give it a try. Then, if you want, get more involved. Because the best thing about a new sport is that it has room for all of us. And that means you, too.

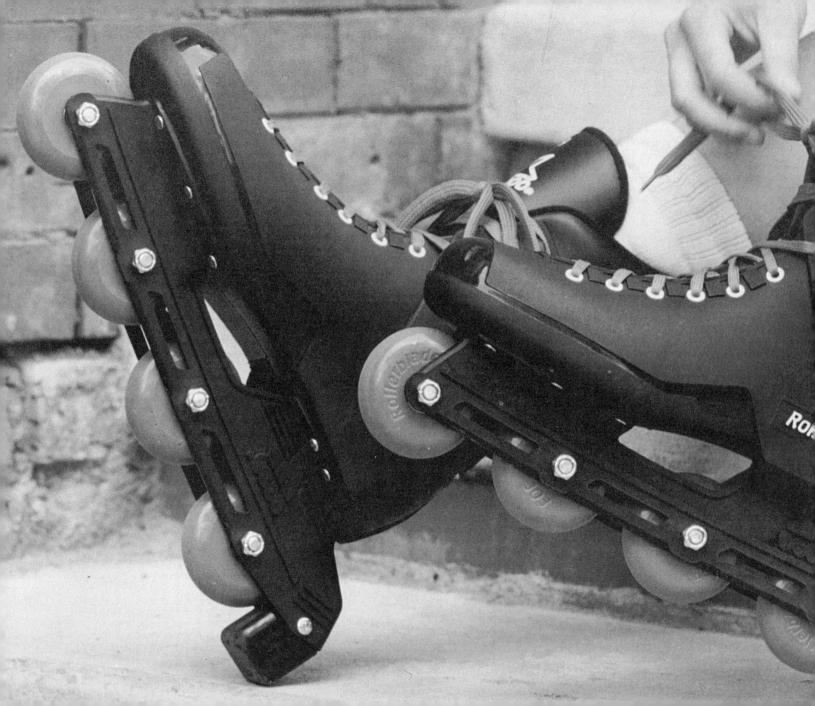

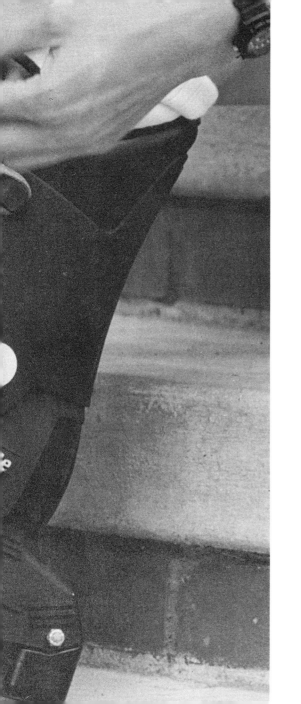

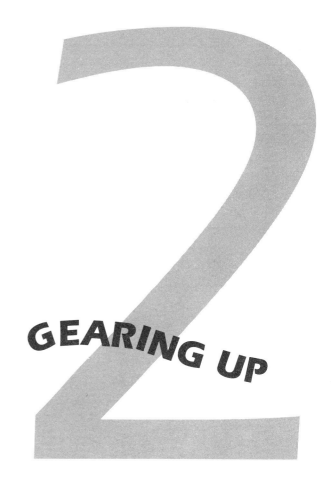

GEARING UP

Before we go any further, we have to talk about buying skates. And before we talk about buying skates, we have to talk about what you expect to get out of them.

Spend a few minutes thinking about yourself, your goals and your personality. Are you an athlete looking for a new sport? Do you get swept up in a new activity easily? Are you competitive? Looking for a workout, or looking for something to do on those sunny weekend afternoons?

The answers will help you choose from the variety of models now available, with price tags from around $100 to over $400. The only way to put the advantages and limitations of various skates into perspective is to know what you expect from them.

If you are athletic and plan to skate for exercise, for instance, you will need a fitness-oriented, high-performance skate. If you plan to enjoy the skates recreationally while talking to your best

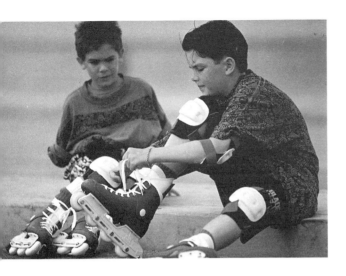

friend, you can get by with a less performance-oriented and less expensive model.

A GOOD FIT

The one criterion that transcends specialization is a good fit. So that you can get one, bring to the store the pair of socks you plan to wear when skating. Many sport or fitness skaters recommend a thin liner sock of silk or polypropylene, which wicks moisture from the foot and cuts down friction between the skate and your foot, worn under a medium-weight athletic sock, which will absorb the excess moisture, or a specially padded athletic sock designed to prevent blisters and moisture buildup. Both types of socks are available at well-stocked sporting goods stores. All-cotton socks, particularly thick ones, don't keep the feet dry and therefore contribute to blisters and other foot problems.

Choose a store that encourages you to spend a few minutes in the skates, and is willing to help you patiently with your questions and concerns. Although it may be difficult to know how the skates will feel once you've been in them for an hour, you should at least feel comfortable in the skates inside the store. If the skates hurt there, you can be sure they will only feel worse on the road.

Like an ice skate or ski boot, an in-line skate boot should fit snugly but allow for a little extra toe room in the front. To check this, put the skates on and stand up with straight knees. Your toes should barely touch but not jam into the front of the boot. Next bend your knees. The action of putting pressure against the front of the boot will cause your toes to drop back. Make sure when they do that that they are not cramped. If they are, the skate is too small.

THE BOOT

Once you have the right size, look for the most breathable boot in your price range. The original in-line skates and many of today's models are made of solid pieces of plastic or polyurethane that don't allow any air to pass to or from the skate. But some boots have vents that allow air circulation. Since feet sweat and then heat up when the air cannot escape, a breathable skate is more comfortable, particularly during long or intense workouts.

Properly positioned vents also improve the fit of the boot, because they allow the skate to conform to the shape of your foot when buckled tight. The vents also make the boot lighter. High-quality vented skates are well worth the additional money if you plan to spend considerable time in them.

Next judge the weight of the skate. A light skate is fast, respon-sive and comfortable. Go to a store that has a number of different models, pick them up and compare. All other things considered, the lighter a skate is, the more fun it will be.

If you are looking for performance, also pay attention to design breakthroughs like the freewheeling, symmetrical hinged cuff. Until recently, the cuff, which is the top part of the skate, was an inflexi-ble part of the boot. Now, however, the hinged cuff with a single ratchet-style buckle provides an extremely efficient forward-flexing combination. A hinged cuff makes it easier to keep your weight forward (which, as you will see, is critical to safe, controlled skating). Because the hinged cuff gives you a more individual fit, it also allows a full range of motion, which is another key to efficient skating. It is such an improvement over the normal cuff, in fact, that it will almost certainly appear soon on the more inexpensive model skates.

You should also pay attention to the boot material, although price may be the determinant here as well. Ideally, you want a boot made of polyurethane, because it is supportive, or of copolymer plastic, which is a state-of-the-art material coming directly out of the Alpine ski industry. If you can help it, though, avoid polyethylene, because it is too flexible to provide sufficient support.

In theory, you should be able to tell "what is what" just by reading the label. Unfortunately, however, a number of companies say their boots are made of polyurethane when they are actually polyethylene. The best way to tell is to take hold of the boot and squeeze it. If it is very pliable or responds to your touch, the material is probably not as good as they claim.

Inside the boot, the key to further comfort and fit is an anatomical insole or foot bed, which noticeably increases shock absorption and provides welcome arch support. The more expensive skates feature liners with memory foam, which conform to your feet and therefore act as a buffer between them and the unforgiving plastic boot. These liners can be bought separately so that you can upgrade the fit and feel of a less expensive skate.

Women with narrow feet should consider purchasing a skate

designed for women's feet—the cuffs are contoured differently and the liners are padded to provide a snug fit for narrow feet.

Because one size of shell can accommodate several different sizes of liners, parents can extend the life of their child's skates by changing the liners as the feet grow.

WHEELS AND BEARINGS

Once you are satisfied with a boot, move on to the wheels and bearings. How many wheels should you have? Most skaters prefer four. If your feet are very small, however, you may have to settle for three, which are slower.

Racers will gravitate toward the racing models, which have five wheels. These skates also excel on hills, thanks to their enhanced edge control. But these remarkable skates, which are very fast and require solid skating technique, were developed with the advanced skater in mind. Unless you have an ice-skating background or are an experienced in-line skater, start with a good, fast four-wheel model.

When checking out wheels, first check the frame upon which they sit. To get a stable ride, you need a rigid frame. Turn the skate over and cradle it in your legs. Then try to twist the frame. If you sense only a slight torque, you can be confident of the skate's support. If it twists, however, it will be unstable. Generally, the most stable frames are made out of nylon with fiberglass reinforcement.

Wheel quality is slightly more complicated, because it depends on diameter (height of wheel), durometer (degree of hardness) and the presence of a core.

Some people mistakenly think that speed is a function only of the durometer. But all three characteristics matter. If you are interested in racing, for instance, you want a high-performance wheel with a large diameter (seventy-six millimeters as compared to sixty-four millimeters for some beginning recreational skates) and a large core. The larger wheels allow a stronger push off and thus more efficient skating, which may make them faster than a smaller, harder wheel.

But maximum speed is usually the goal of only the experienced skater, who has come to prefer a particular wheel through practical experience anyway. If you are a new skater, think about the type of skating you anticipate. If you don't have a lot of money to spend or plan on using the skates only every once in a while, look for the cheaper models of skates, because they traditionally feature a hubless wheel. This makes the wheel smaller in diameter and slower but, as a result, easier to control.

Bearings are similarly designed for various levels of performance. Advanced competitive speed skaters pack their own bearings to make sure they get the maximum advantage. Some skaters who are cross training or working out prefer resistance bearings, which increase friction, forcing them to push harder.

Most skaters, however, want a bearing with a minimum rating of ABEC-1. This is an internationally recognized standard. High-performance racing bearings have an ABEC-5 rating; some of the better recreational bearings have an ABEC-1 rating. Bearings with no ABEC rating are for beginner users and are found on inexpensive skates.

ROCKERING

Some models of in-line skates have an adjustable row of wheels so that you can "rocker" them. When skates come from the factory, they have a flat row of wheels that gives you more stability for most recreational skating and for long, straight skating at increased speeds. By rockering the row of wheels, you can get more maneuverability for quick turns and pivots. Most hockey players, for example, rocker their skates.

To adjust the rocker, remove the middle two wheels from the frame support (or if you have a three-wheeled skate, the middle wheel), using the wrenches provided with your skates. Remove the frame spacers in the holes of the wheel cavity of the frame. Turn the spacers upside down so that the frame will arch out. Both frame spacer openings must be arranged identically so that the axle will fit through. To return the row of wheels to a flat position, reverse the process.

Certain models also have an adjustable wheelbase. Longer bases are best for straight-line stability; shorter lengths, for maneuverability. See the owner's manual for specific instructions.

ROCKERING

The middle two wheels are lower than the two end wheels.

PROTECTIVE GEAR

Once you have decided on the boot, the frame, the wheels, the bearings and the all-important shoe laces, you might think you are done. But don't put away your checkbook yet. Before you leave, throw in a complete set of protective gear.

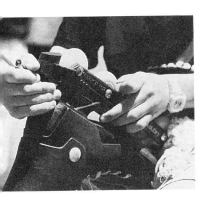

ROTATING THE WHEELS

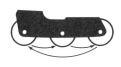

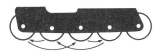

WHEEL ROTATION OF SKATES WITH THREE,
FOUR OR FIVE WHEELS

RISA recommends that all in-line skaters use wrist guards, knee pads, elbow pads and a helmet. Protective gear may seem like just an added expense now, but it may save you a visit to the doctor's office or, worse, the hospital. Although skating is normally a safe activity, it has an element of risk. The safety gear has been developed to protect you from the common skate-related injuries. It is ill-advised to learn without them, or for that matter, to skate without them after you've learned.

If the skater is your child, please be especially sure to buy the proper protective gear and insist on its use every time.

MAINTENANCE

One of the best parts about the skates is that, once you've finally bought them, they are virtually maintenance free. Besides keeping them clean, which can be done by occasionally wiping your skates with a soft, damp cloth, the most important thing you have to do is rotate or reposition the wheels so that they wear evenly.

Even that isn't as difficult or demanding as it used to be. Until 1989, it was thought that the wheels needed to be rotated every sixty or eighty miles. But that advice turned out to be too general. You should rotate the wheels when they begin to wear unevenly and look lopsided.

To rotate them, use an Allen wrench and a socket wrench. (The size depends upon the model of skate, but most high-performance skates use a 5/32-inch Allen wrench and a 7/16-inch socket wrench; most beginning skates, two 1/2-inch wrenches.) For four-wheel skates, the wheel in front (number one) changes places with

27

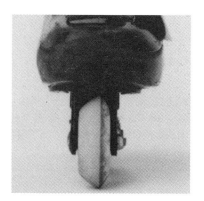

A WORN WHEEL
It should be replaced.

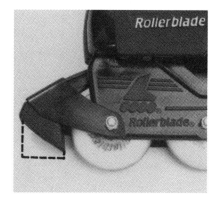

TIME FOR A NEW BRAKE
The dotted line shows its original size.

the wheel that is next to the back (number three); the back wheel (number four) changes with the wheel behind the front (number two). When you replace them, turn each wheel so that the edge with the most wear faces out. Tighten the wheels until there is resistance when you spin them, then use the wrench to back off the setting a bit.

Before you put the wheels back on the skate, take a second to wipe your bearings clean with a soft cloth. They are precision sealed or shielded and therefore need no grease or further care, so long as you stay away from sand, water and rain, which are unsafe both to you and your bearings. If you inadvertently get the skates wet, remove the wheels and towel the bearings off immediately. If you can't, you can wedge a paper towel between the frame and the wheel, spin the wheel and try to dry the bearing.

Except for the brake, you will run through wheels before you run through anything else. Some people trash a set of wheels in a month or two; others take a year. While there is no set time, you will know because they will be slower and less responsive. When it gets to the point that you feel you are fighting them, buy a new set. Bearings, fortunately, last longer.

If you have to tilt your skate to an extreme angle in order to stop, then your brake is probably too worn (see photograph). Replace the brake when its edge is making a 45-degree angle with the street. The replacement procedures vary from model to model, but all are easy to manage.

THE SAFETY CHECK

That's about all there is to it. But just to be on the safe side, get in the habit of doing a safety check every time you get on your skates. To check the axle tightness and the bearings, wiggle each wheel. Then check the nuts that secure the wheels, and make sure they are tight. This is most important just after you change the wheels, but check them out each time anyway. Make sure your brake is not too worn to be effective.

Then strap on your protective gear and get ready to roll.

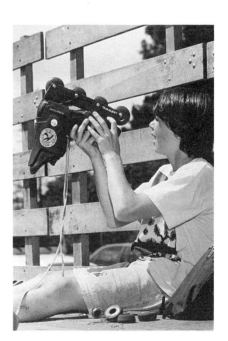

CHECKING THE ALIGNMENT

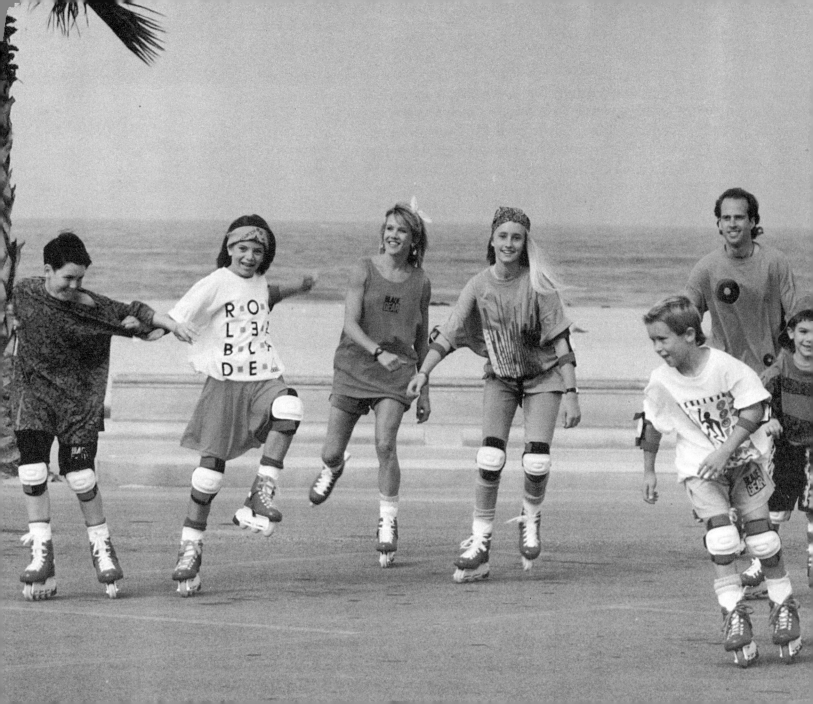

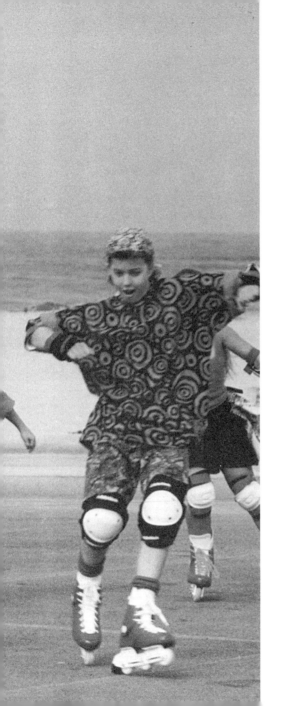

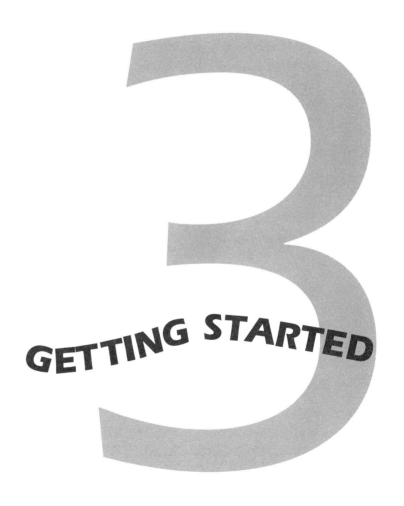

GETTING STARTED

Like beauty, risk is in the eye of the beholder. Some people think nothing of jumping off a high diving board with nothing more than a glance to see that the pool is filled, while others practically have to be lowered in step by step. Yet it is the same dive, with the same water and the same danger level. Only the attitude is different.

Both of these extreme approaches have inherent limitations. While a daredevil is undeniably appealing, leaping before you look can have some nasty consequences. And while the person who sinks slowly into the water does get there eventually, it's only after much unnecessary concern.

Rather than emulate either, you would do well to take a middle ground when learning any new physical skill. With skating, begin by reassuring yourself that people have been learning to skate for centuries—not just athletes, but all kinds of people. If you can walk, you can soon effortlessly skate down the trail.

Sure, you think, that sounds good. But what happens when you encase your feet in boots with wheels and leave solid ground? All the upbeat metaphors, logic and sweet talking don't count for anything beside the terror of losing control and flying down a hill at breakneck speed.

That is, of course, a valid concern, particularly from a beginner's vantage point. But just as there is no reason for casually jumping off a high board without looking, there is absolutely no reason to place yourself in a threatening situation on skates. Until you master the basics, avoid crowds, hills and traffic and take things slowly.

Fortunately, skating can be broken down into several simple and basic skills that are easily and, for most people, quickly learned. Once these skills become second nature, you can work to more advanced terrain, speed or tricks. But that comes later.

ON THE GRASS

For now, think of skating as a walk in the park—literally, as there is no better place to learn balance and control and to develop an initial feel for the skates than a park or grassy area. Since you are trying to give yourself every advantage, choose a level patch of grass, preferably out of the way of bicycles, dogs, nosy pedestrians and baby carriages. Also, since your skates work best when dry and clean, make sure the grass isn't wet or muddy. If you can't find a suitable garden spot, retreat to a carpeted surface indoors, which should provide the same security.

Once you find your spot, lace or buckle your skates so that they are as tight (and thereby as supportive) as possible and get to work. Begin by walking like a duck, with your toes pointed out. This not only gets you used to placing your weight on one foot at a time, but also gets you in the habit of pushing off to the side against the row of wheels. This basic motion will allow you to start to roll immediately.

As you become accustomed to the motion, gradually pick up speed. Continue until you are comfortable enough to run on the skates, but don't go so fast that you can't keep your toes pointed out.

When you are ready for something new, slowly reach over and touch your toes (stretching your hamstrings, the muscles that run down the back of the upper leg). This gives you an idea of how far forward your weight can be on in-line skates, very valuable knowledge when you head out on the pavement.

Once this position becomes comfortable, stand back up and step first on one foot, then the other. Notice how much easier this is when you keep your weight on the inside edge of the skate. Then pay attention to how it feels when you transfer weight from one leg to the other. Practice this until you can jump back and forth from skate to skate. You'll be surprised by how easy it is, and by how eager you will be to take to the pavement.

BASIC STROKING

Choose that first area of concrete carefully. The ideal surface will be flat and well paved. Make sure it is reasonably free of rocks, bumps, potholes, debris and, most importantly, traffic, and that your skates are dry and free of rocks or grass that they might have picked up while off the pavement. Empty parking lots and outdoor tennis or basketball courts are ideal for these first forays.

If you are like most people, the first thing you will want to learn is how to stop. But before you can stop, you have to move. So put the question of stopping aside for a moment and concentrate on your balance. To skate properly, you have to keep your weight on the ball of your foot. The easiest way to do that is to make sure you keep your knees bent at all times.

Bent knees are so important, in fact, that they demand special consideration. When you keep your knees bent, you keep your weight over the skate. This results in much better control, because it keeps you more stable. To understand why, stand up without your skates on. Keep your knees straight, lean slightly back and see how easy it would be for someone to come by and push you over. Then bend your knees, shift your center of gravity forward toward your belly button and you'll see how much harder it would be for someone to throw you off balance.

If you keep your center of gravity above the skates, the wheels are under the body, subject to its power. If you keep your weight on the heels, however, you lose that measure of control. Then, as soon as you lose your balance, the skates go out from under you. As they go out, they tend to propel you backward, making it more likely that you fall in such a way that you injure your tailbone, elbow or head.

(By the way, whenever you learn a new skill—from the basics to stunts—it is a good idea to practice all the motions first without wearing the skates. This enables the body to program itself for the particular movement and may dramatically decrease the time required to learn the skill. It certainly decreases the fear factor.)

While the importance of bent knees seems perfectly logical on paper, most people instinctively stand up straight or even lean back when they're uneasy or afraid. To work against this natural tendency, think about keeping your shin against the tongue of the skate. Although it accomplishes the same result, which is keeping

KEEP THE KNEES BENT

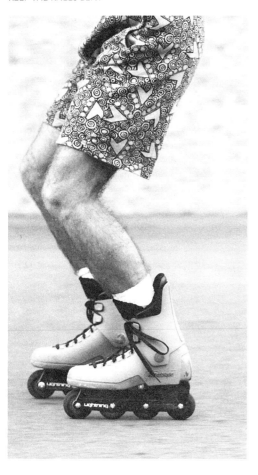

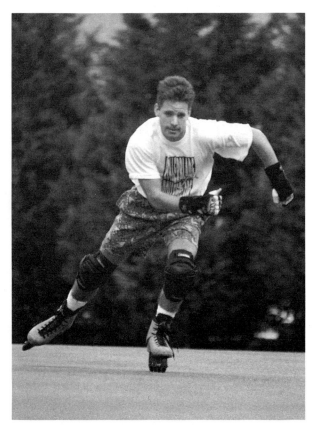

STROKING WITH GOOD FORM

the weight on the balls of the feet and the center of gravity forward, it is an easier image to visualize than bent knees for most people.

Once you get the hang of this stance, you are ready to start skating. For stability, keep your hands low and in front of you—wild or uncontrolled arm motions will only throw off your balance. Push off with one leg, going as far out to the side—as opposed to the back—as you can. Since that leg is in the air, concentrate on keeping all your weight on the opposite leg, which will give you power and stability, and on keeping the standing knee bent.

To get the most out of each stride, push with the entire row of wheels. Envision all the wheels on the ground, and pushing from that surface. After you have pushed out the leg as far as you can, bring it back to center, transfer your weight onto it and push out with the opposite leg. Do it a few times and you're skating!

STOPS

Up to this point, everything is all well and good. But all good things must come to an end, or, in this case, a stop. And for many people, that is the most difficult part of in-line skating.

Since there are several ways to stop, however, it should not be a problem. Because it takes some time to become proficient at fast stops, though, it may help at first if you think in terms of slowing down rather than of stopping on a dime.

Although stopping is not a difficult maneuver, it can be tricky at first. Be safe, not sorry, by always exercising caution: Never skate on terrain or locations that are too difficult or crowded for you, and brake before, not after, you get out of control.

Perhaps the most common way to stop is with the heel brake. (If you are used to conventional roller skates, continually remind yourself that in-line skates do not have toe stops.) With this method, all you have to do is bend forward at the waist and scissor the leg with the brake forward until the brake is parallel to the front wheel of the other skate. Tilt the foot with the heel stop up and exert pressure by bending your knee. The more pressure you place on the brake, the quicker you will stop.

The second method of stopping is called the T-stop. Keep one foot forward, with the skate pointed straight ahead and the knee bent. Slightly lift your other foot, move it behind you and, keeping a bent knee, place it perpendicular to the front foot (or in an inverted T position). Then lower the rear skate to the ground. With the knee slightly bent, drag the inner edge of your wheels while pressing downward. Hold your feet firmly to the ground, and use the inner thigh for strength and stability. Although more difficult than the basic stop, this is a much flashier move.

Since today's wheels are designed for abrasive use, don't worry about doing them any damage. But since the T-stop is more difficult than the heel brake, work on it at slower speeds until you are confident of your ability. Then, if you want to get really fancy, work on an advanced T-stop, in which you drag only the back toe of the skate.

There is a third way to stop—by slowing down until you do a controlled 360-degree turn with your feet turned out. This movement will reduce your speed and effectively bring you to a halt. To

STOPPING WITH THE BRAKE

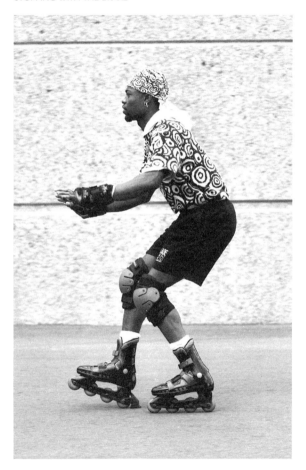

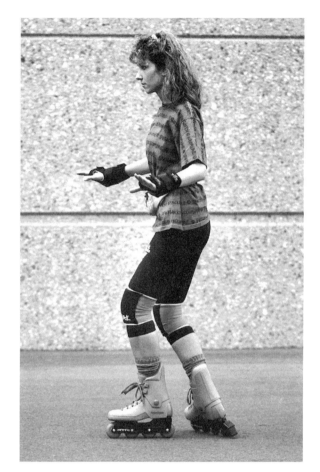

A T-STOP

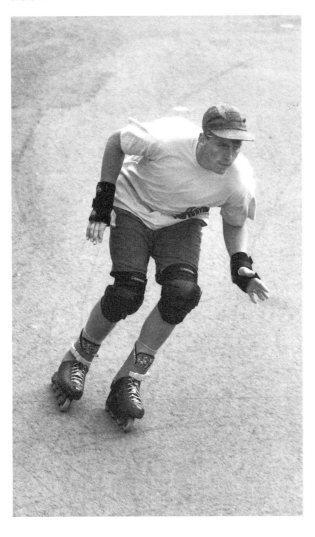

keep the movement steady, you should control any arm and upper body movements.

Finally, there is the power stop, an advanced move which we'll describe in the rollerhockey chapter as it's used almost exclusively in that game.

TURNS

Now pay attention to turning. If you are a skier, you have a head start because turns on skates are very similar to turns on skis. Both require edge control and angulation, which is a fancy term for being able to lean on the inside of the skate. To turn, you must shift your weight so you're on the edge of the wheels. The more weight you can place on the edge, the more responsive the skate will be on the turn.

To turn to the left, place your weight on the inside edge of your right foot. As you do, bend the knee to increase the force on the edge. This makes the skate more responsive and enables you to turn more quickly.

Complete the turn by pointing your hands and knees in the direction you want to go. Throughout, keep the bend in your knees and thighs, and point the hands from the elbow rather than the shoulders. Remember that in-line skates are extremely responsive. Rather than exaggerate the motion, you will do much better with smaller, more controlled moves.

While this type of turn serves for basic conditions, more experienced skaters prefer a second type of turn, called a crossover, which allows you to maintain and even increase your speed. First, find a flat surface. You might consider putting a cone or some other visible object on the pavement to help you turn at a specific point.

First practice by stepping the right foot over the left, and the left over the right. Repeat this movement until you feel comfortable.

It is easier to do crossovers if you get some speed first, because you are going to have to use the outside edge to complete the turn. If you go too slowly, you have to fight inertia, which makes the movement more difficult.

Start with your stronger side. For most people, that will be the right over the left. (To compensate, spend extra time practicing on the weaker side—since most skating routes involve at least one of each, this will come in handy once you get on the road.)

For a right-over-left crossover, first hold the outside edge of the left skate and cross over, or step through, on the right foot, using the inside edge of the right wheels. To help ensure stability, keep your hands out in front of you, shoulder width apart. Look ahead into the turn and keep looking at it as you begin making the turn. This should help you commit to making the turn. Then push away with the left foot and complete the maneuver by bringing the leg back to center.

SKATING BACKWARD

Skating backward on in-line skates is not difficult. Perhaps the most difficult part, in fact, is believing that it is both fun and within your ability.

As with any other skill, the best way to gain confidence is by

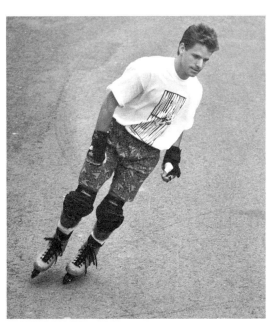

CROSSOVER TURN   1

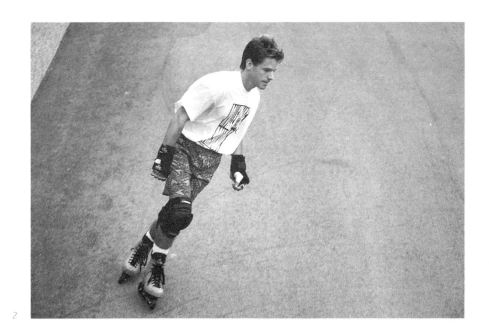

2

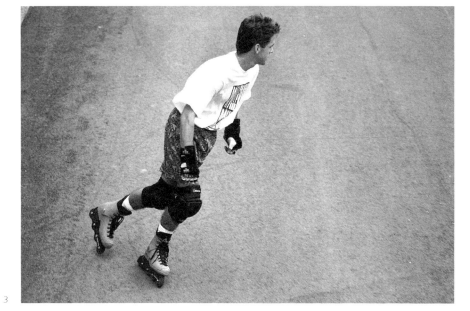

3

starting slowly. First find a flat surface. Keep the knees slightly bent and the feet under the shoulders. Pigeon the toes of the feet in and keep the knees together. Push out by keeping the weight on the inside edges, and swizzle both feet until each one is beyond the shoulder. Keeping the inside edge, use the strength of the inside thighs to bring the heels together and back to position one. Repeat and build up speed by becoming slightly more aggressive with your moves.

Before you can learn backward crossovers, you have to learn how to place most of your weight on one foot. Keeping both feet on the ground, push off on the inside edge of your stronger foot. As you do, lean on the outside edge of the other skate. Bring the leg back in so that it is parallel with the other and so that both feet are directly under your shoulders. Your weight is mostly on your stronger foot. Then repeat with the other foot.

To learn backward crossovers, work on a smooth area that has a slight curve to make it easier to build momentum. Skate backward until you hit a moderate speed. While on the curve, place your weight on the left foot's back outside edge. Using the right back inside edge, cross the right foot over. Then lift or pull the left leg up and replace it in the same place the right foot used to be. (If you favor the other foot, reverse the directions.) During the move, the right foot should barely, if at all, leave the ground.

Staying on course may be easier if you visualize going around the painted lines of an imaginary circle (or find a real circle on an outdoor basketball court). Keep your arms straight over the line, one in front of you and one in back—and your shoulders and chest facing inside the circle. And look over your shoulder in the direction you are going.

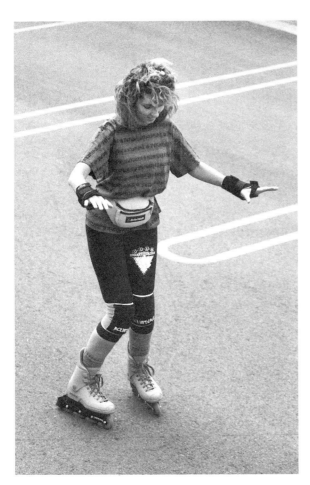

SWIZZLING BACKWARD   1

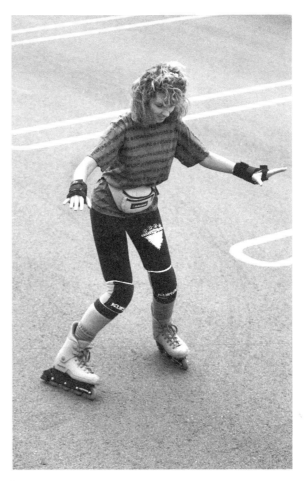

2

43

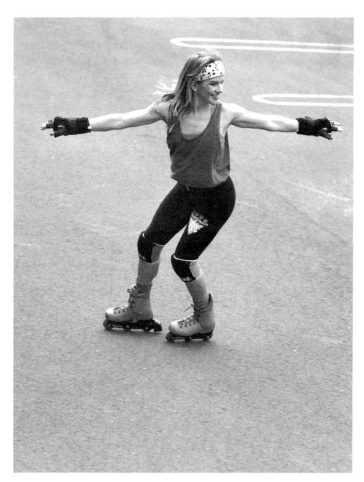

BACKWARD CROSSOVER 1

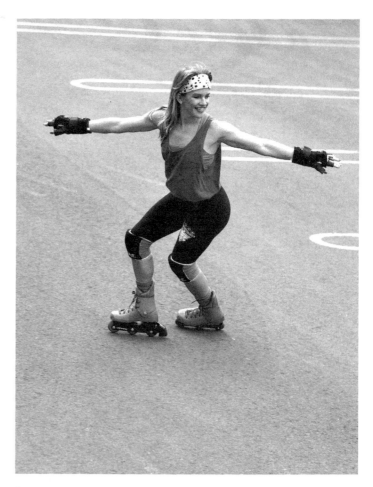

2

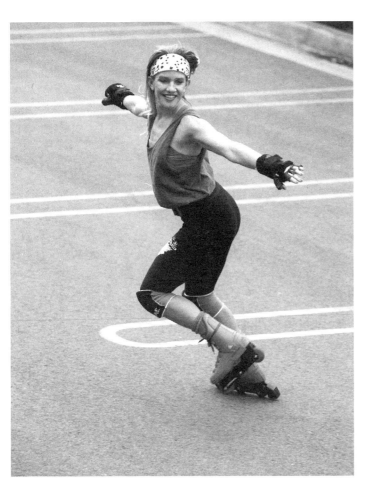

3

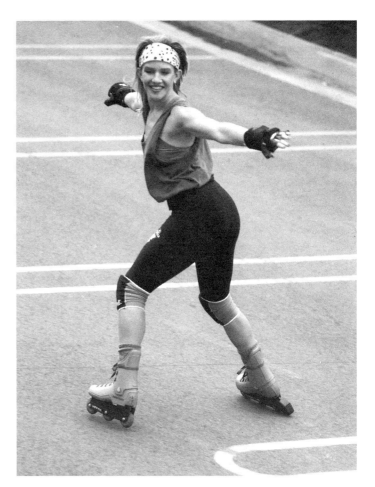

4

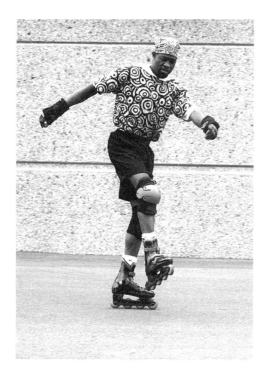

TURNING FROM FORWARD TO BACKWARD SKATING 1

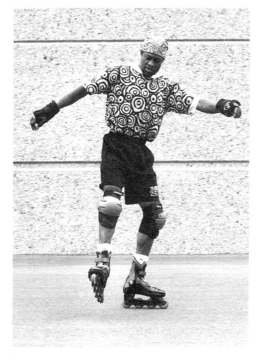

2

3

GETTING STARTED

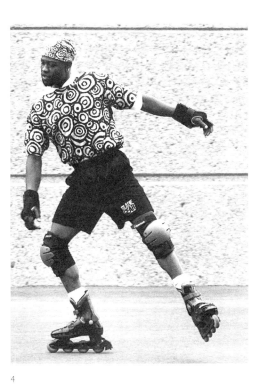

The transition from forward to backward skating (or vise versa) is considerably easier. Go back to a flat surface and skate forward in a straight line. Place your weight on your left foot, and step forward on the right inside edge. As you do, open the left shoulder out. This will start you turning to the left. As you continue the turn, step back on the left inside edge so that it is turned out. Lift the toe of the right foot slightly and let it come down as the body turns completely backward. When the turn is complete, step on the forward left skate's flat frame edge, push off and continue your stroke. And have a little trust. This is a fluid, fast move that sounds a lot more complicated than it really is.

Once you have these basic skills, you are ready to diversify. Will it be racing, stunts, hockey or fitness skating for you—or maybe all of them?

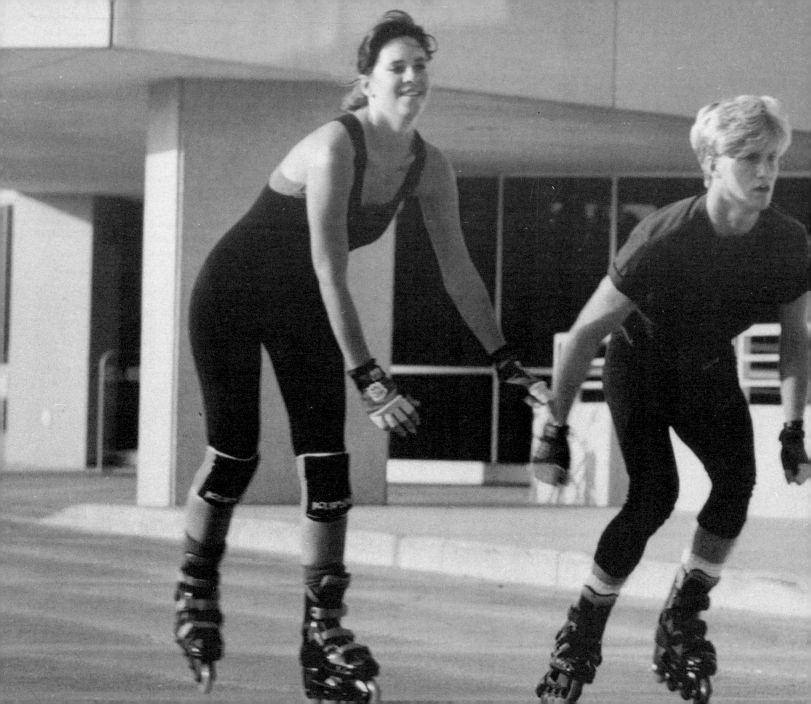

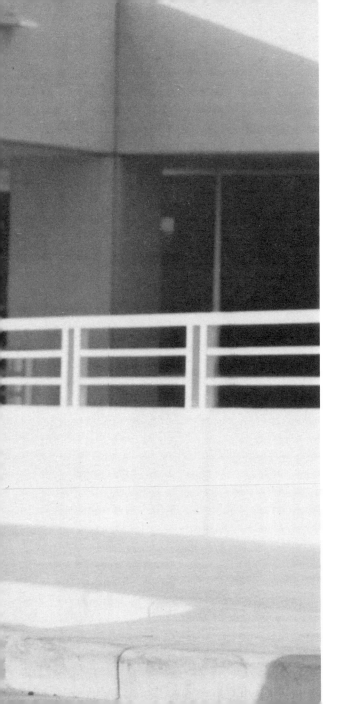

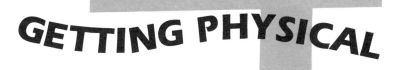

4
GETTING PHYSICAL

As you already know, skating is one of the most effective low-impact activities. It can be the cornerstone of any fitness program, because it conditions the cardiopulmonary system without placing a dangerous amount of stress on the muscles and joints.

Results of a recent fitness study, testing the effectiveness of in-line skating as a cardiovascular activity, conclusively demonstrated what skaters and other athletes have known all along: In-line skating compares favorably to running, cycling and other training regimens.

According to the study, which was conducted by Carl Foster, Ph.D., associate professor of medicine at the University of Wisconsin Medical School and coordinator of sports medicine and sports science for the United States Speed Skating Team, recreational in-line skaters burn 285 calories during a thirty-minute skate. (Proficient speed skaters can burn about 450 calories during the same time.) Although this is less than the 350 and 360 calories runners and cyclists burn, even recreational skaters fall well within the 300 calories/workout guidelines established by the American College of Sports Medicine.

In addition, skating places less impact on the musculoskeletal system than running, greatly reducing the risks of injury associated with the pounding of the hip, knee, ankle and foot joints. In-line

HEART RATE TARGET (TEN-SECOND COUNT)

Safe training zone equals 70 to 80 percent of maximum heart rate

Age	55%	60%	70%	80%	85%
15	19	21	24	27	29
20	18	20	23	27	28
25	18	19	23	26	28
30	17	19	22	25	27
35	17	19	22	25	26
40	17	18	21	24	26
45	16	18	20	23	25
50	16	17	20	23	24
55	15	17	19	22	23
60	15	16	19	21	23
65	14	16	18	21	22

FROM THE AMERICAN HEART ASSOCIATION

skating develops the hip and knee extensor (thigh) muscles that are not well developed by running or cycling. It also works the hamstring, which is not strengthened by cycling. So in-line skating is superior at toning the lower body muscles.

YOUR TRAINING ZONE

As with any workout, however, you have to do more than just put on a pair of skates and effortlessly stroll around the neighborhood. Instead you have to skate long and hard enough to push your heart rate into its training zone (see chart). Before starting any new fitness program, consult with a physician. After you get the go-ahead, exercise at a pace you would consider moderate to somewhat strenuous—more will actually do more harm than good. The chart will help you find your safe training zone, which is between 70 to 80 percent of your maximum heart rate.

Another way to figure out your maximum heart rate is to subtract your age from 220. To find your training zone, multiply the maximum heart rate by .7. The last number you need to know is that, after cooling down, your heartbeat should be under 100 beats a minute.

THE ROLLERBLADE 30-MINUTE WORKOUT™

Before you can work out effectively, you have to be able to skate at a continuous and relatively intense pace for at least twenty minutes. You also have to find a place where you can keep up the pace without interruptions. A bike path is often ideal; a very large parking lot will do. Streets with traffic, stop lights and signs are not recommended. Not only are they unsafe, but your workout will be interrupted. Since the body recovers in much less than a minute, these delays interfere with the effectiveness of the workout.

Once you have the necessary skills and location, you must approach skating as you would any other conditioning activity. If all you want are the cardiopulmonary benefits, you need to skate only about twenty minutes three times a week.

If your goal is weight control and stress management, you may want to skate between four and six times a week at a moderately intense pace for forty-five to sixty minutes. Although in-line skating is too new to have developed strict standards for avoiding overuse injuries, the low-impact nature of the sport suggests that these distances are well within the safety range.

For those who have a limited amount of time, or who may have trouble maintaining the speed required for a high-intensity aerobic workout of twenty to thirty minutes, Dr. Foster has developed a Rollerblade 30-Minute Workout™, which will develop your cardiovascular (aerobic) fitness level while strengthening the muscles of the lower legs.

A person wanting a general fitness workout should skate a slow warm-up for five minutes, skate at a comfortable, steady pace for twenty minutes and skate a slow cooldown for five minutes. Data suggest that a person following this workout can increase aerobic power 15 to 20 percent and burn 14,000 calories by skating three to four times a week for three months.

A serious fitness participant or competitive athlete should

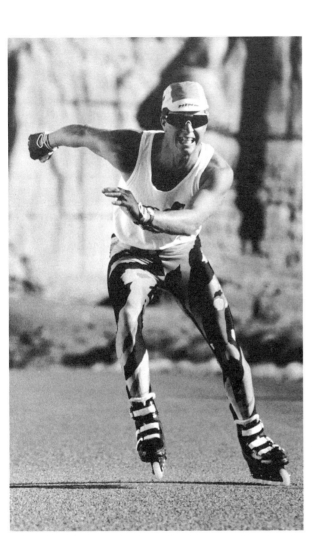

skate a slow warm-up for five minutes, then skate in one-minute intervals for twenty minutes, alternating skating in a standing position and in a tuck position. As the workout becomes comfortable, spend more time in the tuck position to work the hip and knee extensor muscles. Data suggest that a person following this workout can burn 20,000 calories by skating three to four times a week for three months.

Because athletes can reach a higher aerobic limit through hard cycling or running than by in-line skating on level ground, in-line skaters looking for the maximum aerobic workout should use uphill courses. They should first master the techniques of hill climbing in the chapter about extreme skating and should always use caution when going downhill.

Regardless of the intensity of the workout, take off your skates afterward and gently stretch the major muscle groups you have used. Do the calf stretch, hamstring stretch, quad stretch and hip stretch described below, holding each stretch for at least thirty seconds. By doing so, you will hasten the muscles' recovery time and protect yourself from injury.

WARMING UP AND COOLING DOWN

Whether you are skating twenty minutes three times a week or an hour a day, it is very important to begin and end the workout properly. When you don't take the time to warm up, you get tired and winded faster and dramatically increase your risk of injury.

Because warming up is so easy, there is no reason to incur these problems. All you have to do is skate at a slower speed for

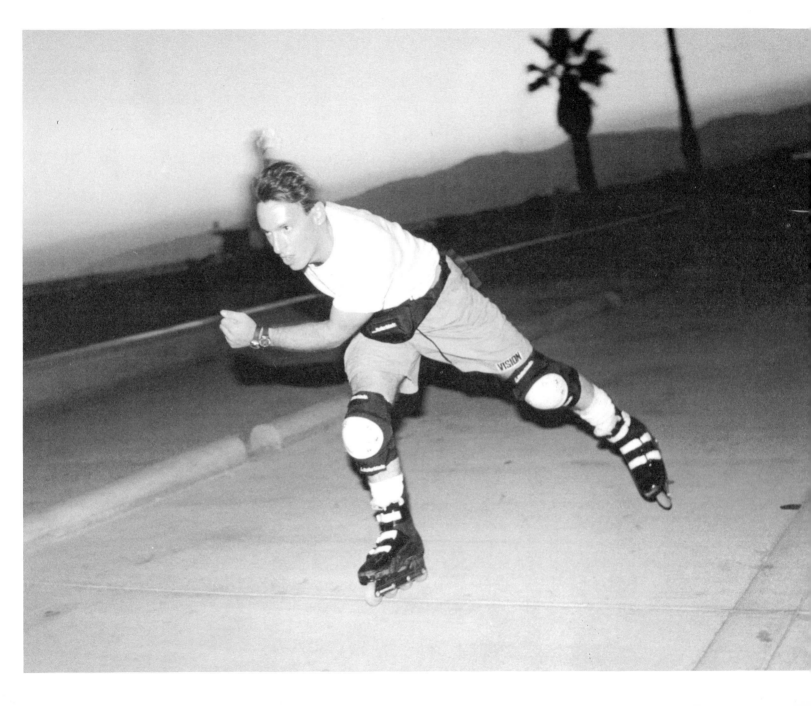

the first five minutes of the workout. Gradually increase the effort until you are just about to break into a sweat. This painless warm-up gets the blood flowing into the legs and prepares the body for the workout.

Besides not warming up at all, one of the biggest mistakes you can make is stretching to warm up. To understand why, think of the muscles as pieces of taffy. If you try to pull apart cold taffy, it breaks in two, leaving tiny, jagged edges. Warm taffy, on the other hand, can be pulled and stretched without ripping.

Similarly, when the body muscles are cold, as they are before an exercise session, stretching can cause microscopic muscle tears. Once muscles are warmed up and have blood flowing in them, they are much more elastic.

For that reason, you should never stretch at the beginning of the workout. If you feel extremely tight, spend five minutes walking around at a moderate pace so that the body is warmed up. At that point, you may safely stretch. Or you can save the stretches for the end of the workout, when they are most effective.

After you have completed the aerobic portion of your workout, slow down the pace. Within five minutes, your breathing and heart rate should return to the normal range. At that point, take your skates off and stretch the most important muscle groups. Some of the most effective exercises are detailed in the workout below.

STRENGTH AND FLEXIBILITY EXERCISES

To increase your performance on in-line skates, as well as develop general fitness, do the following exercises two or three times a week. These exercises have been developed specifically to

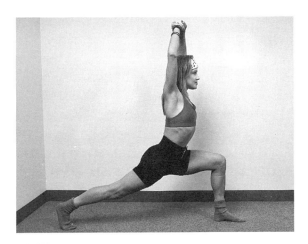

LUNGES

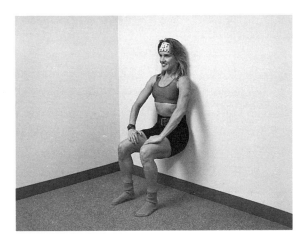

WALL SITS

strengthen and protect the muscles you need to in-line skate well.

The routine can be done in less than half an hour; requires no special equipment; and works the lower back, the abdominal (stomach) muscles, the gluteus (buttocks) and hip muscles and the various muscles in the legs, including the hamstrings, quadriceps, calves and Achilles tendon.

Because the legs are so important, we start with them. Then, because skating also makes demands on the lower back, there are exercises to increase lower-back strength and flexibility. Some of these work the abdominals, because lower-back strength and safety rely on abdominal strength. Anyone who skates regularly will benefit by doing the back and abdominal exercises three to four times a week.

Unless otherwise indicated, hold each stretch for twenty to sixty seconds, and repeat each strength-training exercise until mild fatigue forces you to lose your form and control.

To prevent injuries and hasten recovery time, ease into the stretch. Never go into it too deeply or quickly, and back off at the first sign of pain. Stretching is done to give the body a chance to relax, not to put further stress on it.

Lunges

Step forward, making sure the toe of your front leg is in front of your knee. In a controlled motion, settle down into the lunge position. As you do, make sure your toe and knee remain lined up. Using your quadriceps, hamstring and gluteus muscles, hold the lunge for several seconds. Then push back, return to a neutral position and repeat with the opposite leg. For an advanced version,

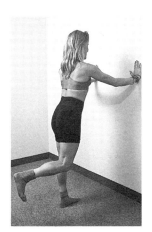
LEG EXTENSIONS AND
LEG CURLS

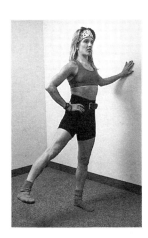
HIP STRENGTHENER

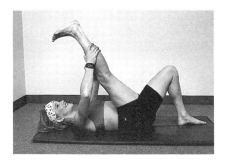
HAMSTRING STRETCH

hold a five- to ten-pound weight in each hand and keep your arms at your sides. Or hold your arms above your head. Repeat twelve to fifteen times on each side, if possible.

Wall sits
Stand against a wall and press your lower back into it. Slide down until your hamstrings are almost parallel to the ground. Place your hands on your upper legs. Hold for twenty to ninety seconds. If the position is too difficult, drop your arms to your sides.

For an advanced version, face a rail, bar or wall. Place the toe behind the heel and go into a one-legged squat.

Leg extensions and leg curls
Stand about two feet from a wall, facing it. Lightly touching the wall for balance, lift one leg to a 90-degree angle. Keep the foot flexed, the pelvis tucked and the buttocks muscles tight. Add resistance by keeping the leg bent at this angle and doing slow pulses. Add more resistance by tightening the buttocks. Repeat until you are mildly fatigued, then repeat with the opposite leg.

Hip strengthener
Stand against a wall for balance. With one hand on your hip, flex the opposite foot and raise it. Point, flex and lower it with control until you are mildly fatigued. Repeat with the opposite leg.

Hamstring stretch
While on your back on the floor, bend one leg so that your foot is against the knee of the other leg, which is extended. Raise the

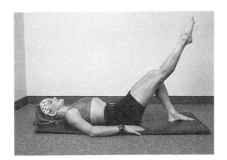

LEG RAISES

extended leg, making sure to keep the feet relaxed. Put your hands on your calf or as high up on the extended leg as you can and pull it towards you. To intensify the stretch, flex your foot. Repeat with the other leg.

Leg raises

Lie on your back with your knees bent. Make sure your lower back is in constant contact with the mat. Keeping the legs parallel, slowly extend one leg. Keep the leg of the extended foot pointed; hold it up for a moment and lower it with control. Alternate legs, and do between twelve and fifteen repetitions if possible.

Afterward, repeat the exercise, supporting yourself on your elbows this time.

Next turn out both feet slightly. Lift the leg straight up until you feel a slight pull in the inner thigh.

Calf raises

Balance yourself, facing a wall. Standing about two feet from it, with your toes out, pelvis tucked in and feet apart, lift up on your toes. Lower with control.

Calf stretch

Stand about two feet from a wall. Place your hands on the wall. Step one foot back about three feet. With the pelvis tucked and knee bent, bend forward until you feel a stretch in the calf muscle. As an option, you can place both legs out and alternate feet, pushing down and stretching the muscle as if you were walking but not moving your feet.

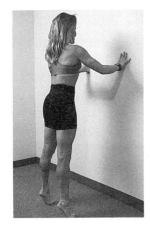

CALF RAISES

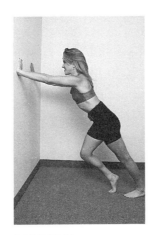

CALF STRETCH

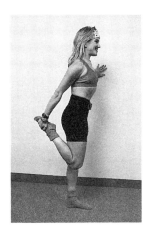

QUAD STRETCH

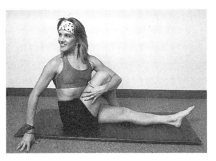

HIP STRETCH

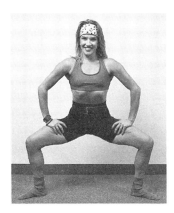

INNER THIGH STRENGTHENER

Quad stretch

Hold on to a chair, pole or table for balance. Grasp your shin and pull your foot back toward your buttocks until you feel the stretch in the quadriceps. Hold and then repeat with the other leg.

Hip stretch

Sit up on the floor. Extend one leg and point the foot. Cross your other leg in front of you. Place your arm across the crossed knee. With your back straight, look around and gently pull the knee until you feel the stretch in the hip of the extended leg. Hold and repeat with the other leg.

Inner thigh strengthener

Stand with feet slightly wider than shoulder width apart, toes pointing out and knees slightly bent. Tuck the pelvis under and place your hands on your thighs for support. Squeeze your buttock muscles and thighs, and sink down to almost a right angle or until you feel a slight stretch in the inner thigh. Repeat until you are mildly fatigued.

Outer thigh strengthener (not pictured)

Hop from one leg to another, pretending you are jumping over an imaginary line.

Upper abdominal curls

Lying on your back with your feet on the ground, shoulder width apart, and your knees bent, press your lower back into the floor. Keep your hands behind your head and your elbows behind you.

59

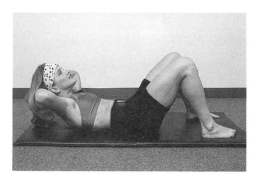

UPPER ABDOMINAL CURLS

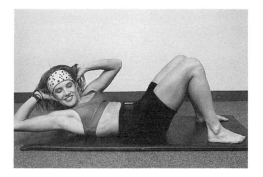

ALTERNATE OBLIQUE CURLS

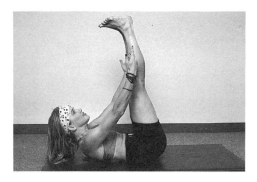

EXTENDED FOOT CURL

Without using your hands to pull you up, curl up 30 degrees. Make sure the lower back remains pressed to the mat. Slowly lower, and repeat until you are mildly fatigued.

Alternate oblique curls
Assume the same starting position as for the upper abdominal curl. Try to reach the opposite side of your body, making sure to feel the twist in the oblique (side) muscles of the abdomen. Slowly return to starting position and repeat until you are mildly fatigued. Do not start the twist too early on the ascent. You may either do one side and then the other or alternate sides.

Extended foot curls
Lie down on your back. With your lower back pressed to the floor, lift your legs toward the ceiling. With your feet flexed, lift the upper body and reach for your toes, making sure that the lower back remains on the floor and that the motion originates from the abdominal muscles. Lower with control. Repeat until you are mildly fatigued.

Note: There are many other equally effective exercises that strengthen the abdominals. Feel free to substitute, but make sure that you include exercises for the three major abdominal muscle groups: the upper and lower abdomen muscles (rectus abdominus, which allow bending forward and sideways at the spine, control in the tilt of the pelvis and consequently influence the curvature of the lower spine) and the internal and external obliques, which make rotation to the right and left possible.

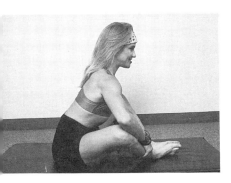

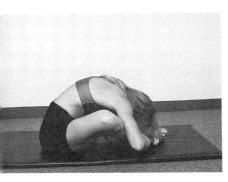

BACK STRETCH

Back stretch

Sit comfortably on the floor with your feet out in front of you. Place your hands on your shins. Keeping your lower back straight, pull directly forward. You should feel the stretch in the hip flexors and lower back.

After you have held this stretch, slide your hands to your ankles, but not to your toes. Pull yourself slightly forward so that the back rounds and you feel the stretch in the entire back.

UPPER-BODY EXERCISES

If you use skating as the cornerstone of your fitness program, you should also incorporate some sort of upper-body exercise, such as swimming or weight training, into your routine.

There are numerous weight-training routines available. Here are some basic exercises that, done two or three times a week, will give the major muscles of the upper body a good workout.

Half-shoulder flies (shoulder muscles)

Stand with your feet straight ahead, shoulder width apart, and your knees directly over your toes. Slightly bend your knees, tuck your buttocks in, pull your stomach in tight and keep your back straight. Slowly lift the weights out to the sides, as close to shoulder height as possible. Lower the arms slowly with control until your palms touch the sides of your body. Don't arch the back in this or any other strengthening exercise. If you can't lift the weight without arching your back, use a lighter weight or do the exercise without weights.

Pullbacks (back of shoulder, latissimus, triceps)
Keeping the same basic stance, begin with the weights at your sides. Exhale as you slowly pull your arms back to an extended position. Pause slightly at the point of maximal extension, and return your arms to the starting position in a controlled manner.

Upright rows (upper chest, biceps, shoulders, upper back)
This exercise requires a barbell loaded with a manageable amount of weight. Stand with your feet shoulder width apart, knees slightly bent, buttocks tucked under, stomach pulled tight. Your arms should hang straight down, and your head should be in a neutral position. Place your hands three to four inches apart over the bar. Exhale as you pull the bar up to your chin. Maintaining the same stance, lower the bar back to just below your waist and repeat until you are mildly fatigued.

Bicep curls
Do this exercise either with free weights or a barbell. Assume a neutral stance and hold the bar or weight with an undergrip. If you use a bar, the hands should be one to three inches apart. Tuck your elbows in and begin with your arms fully extended but not locked. Curl the weight to chest height, keeping your elbows in contact with your upper torso at all times. Lower with control.

Dumbbell bench press (triceps, chest, front shoulder)
Sit down on the bench in a straddle position. The weights should be on the floor, one by each side of the bench, parallel to your hands. Lean down and pick up the weights. Then gently ease yourself onto your back. Keep the elbows bent. Lying on your

back, exhale as you lift the weights. As you do, roll them inward so that your palms face each other at the top of the movement. Then slowly rotate and lift the weights so that they again face outward. Take care not to lock your elbows on the descent as well.

Tricep dips (chest, shoulders, triceps)
With bent elbows and arms pushed back, place both your palms on top of a bench, clasping your fingers on the edge for support or leverage. Extend your legs out. Keep the weight on the heels and your toes up. Slowly straighten your arms and lift yourself up in the air until you have straight but not overextended elbows. As you exhale, bend the elbows and lower yourself until the buttocks nearly touch the ground. Inhale, lift and repeat until you are mildly fatigued.

Chin-ups and push-ups
The good old basics.

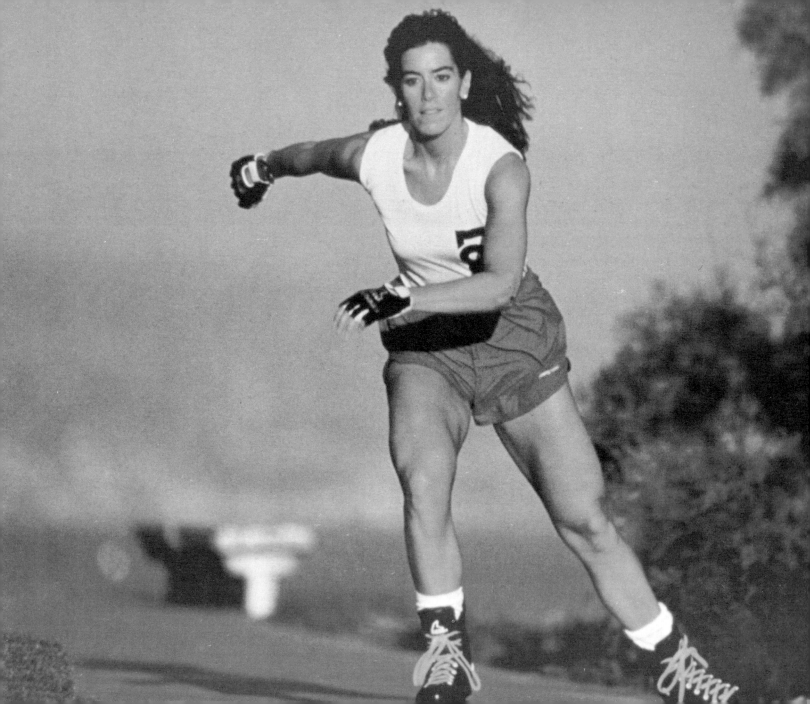

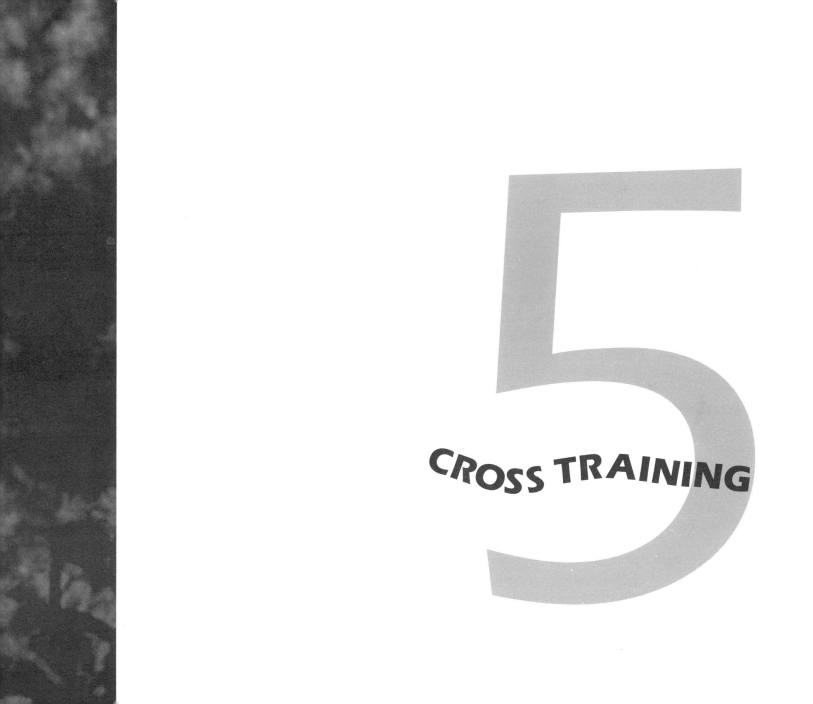

5
CROSS TRAINING

In-line skates were originally developed for ice-hockey players who wanted to keep in shape in the off-season. Although skating has gone way beyond that original vision, many people still use in-line skating in cross training.

HOW IN-LINE SKATING HELPS

Jay Thorson has said that in-line skates "indirectly led to my best year as a decathlete. The skating gives me a good aerobic workout without the pounding that running gives. You have to use many different muscles in the decathlon, and in-line skating forces you to use many more of these muscles than a normal running workout does." Skating also vastly improved his balance, and strengthened his lower back, which improved his distance in the throwing events.

Sports such as snowboarding and surfing are compatible because skating helps to build balance and a strong lower back. Snowboarder Kevin Delaney says, "In-line skating is like snowboarding in that you get the feeling of being airborne and having to shift your body to perform tricks. It helps my balance, which is a critical

virtually every other sport results in a higher level of overall fitness, mental freshness and even performance. While the interplay between in-line skating and these other sports increases overall fitness, in-line skating plays the most specific role in cross-training regimens for skiing, hockey and ice skating. Not only do these sports use the same muscles, but specific skills translate directly from one discipline to the other.

For example, National Hockey League star Luc Robitaille credits much of his success to off-season in-line skating. Because there is little difference between in-line skating and ice-hockey skating, players don't have to make special adjustments to their skating workout before it can make them better hockey players.

SKIING

Ed Pitoniak, an editor at *SKI* magazine, says, "The snowless season—some people call it summer—used to drive me nuts, but in-line skates have made it a lot more bearable.

"I skate more for leg strength than for aerobic training,"Pitoniak reports. "Skates are the best tool I know for building the butt and thigh power you need for good skiing." He continues, "In-line skates also allow me to work on a lot of the fine points of skiing during the off-season. Good skiing is essentially the art of balancing on one leg while riding a narrow edge of steel around an arc. Balance and edge angles are the keys here, and skates allow you to work on both."

In a typical session, he'll cruise on flats, skate up hills hard and work on his turns going downhill. He also works on keeping his upper body quiet, and on practicing certain skills.

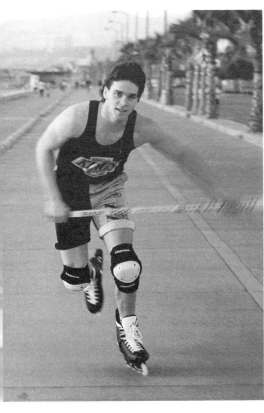

NHL STAR LUC ROBITAILLE

Even so, he does not consider it primarily a workout. "I skate mainly to have fun. But the great thing about skates is that you can go out just planning to rip around, and still get great conditioning and technical benefits."

In-line skates have become such a popular cross-training method for skiers that Rollerblade, Inc. produced a "Skate to Ski" video with the help of the Professional Ski Instructors of America and the United States Ski Team.

While any skating program can improve skiing skills, serious skiers can dramatically improve their performance with some specific exercises on skates.

Sprinting and slaloming down hills, for instance, use the same muscles on skates as on skis. Start on a slight incline. To simulate gates, set cans or other markers about fifteen feet apart. Make sure to allow for a considerable run-out at the end of the course. If you can, make the exercise truly sports specific by using ski poles with carbide tips.

To hone your turns, shift your weight from foot to foot and toe to toe, just as you would on skis. Initiate the turn with your weight on the ball of your outside foot, and then sink down into the turn. As you come up, drive your weight onto the heel. To complete the turn, transfer your weight onto the opposite foot.

Continue turning until you get down the incline. Throughout, remember to keep your body pointed downhill. Instead of turning the shoulders, keep them square to the hill. Your arms should be in front of you for balance, and your center of gravity should always be in the abdomen.

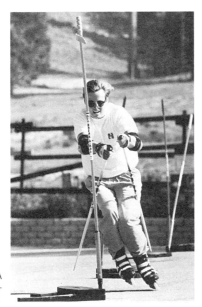

SLALOMING AROUND A GATE WITH PROPER POLING TECHNIQUE 1

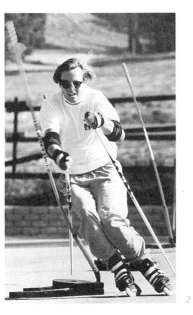

2

When the incline becomes too easy, intensify the exercise either by moving to a steeper incline or spreading the gates farther apart, up to eight feet.

If, on the other hand, the incline is too difficult, practice turning on level ground without any markers. Build up speed, then carve turns for as long as you can. Build up some more speed and carve away again.

Although some nonskiing skaters have toyed with the idea of using poles as a way to involve the upper body in a general fitness program, poles have mostly been used in the slalom and for Nordic (cross-country) skiers who want to improve their timing and stride.

When using a pole, select one that goes under your armpit and slightly pushes your shoulders up when you are on skates. Either a Nordic pole with a carbide tip or a special skating pole will work on asphalt or blacktop. Neither, however, will be able to grip cement.

There are three techniques Nordic skiers can replicate on skates to improve their timing and skiing. The first, which is called V-1, requires the skater to push and pole on the same leg. Just after you start the push, begin to pole. Bring it up so that the tip hits at the heel of the skate. Although you can use a little arm swing, do not flex the arm or move it in front. Get the arm back to full extension as you finish the push. Then, before you begin again, make sure to glide. Stay on the inside edge or, to simulate the motion more closely, start with a level row of wheels and move to the inside edge.

To work on a more competitive, faster stroke, do what is called the V-2, which is a pattern of three pushes with a poling motion on the third. Unlike the first exercise, you also switch legs each time.

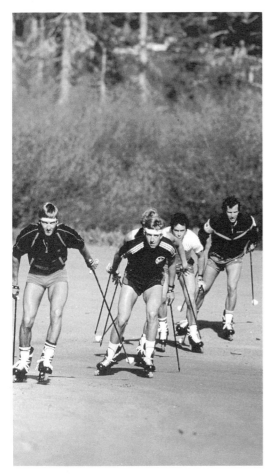

NORDIC SKI TRAINING

The final technique is double poling. As the name implies, you use both poles at the same time. In double poling, you don't move the legs or feet. Rather than flex at the waist, as it is commonly pictured, stand upright and keep the abdominal and buttock muscles tight. This is, obviously, an excellent upper-body workout.

Because improper use of the pole can result in tendinitis of the wrist, elbow or shoulder and can also lead to your being skewered by the blunt end of a pole, proper pole technique is very important. Never angulate the poles or the arms. Instead, keep them slightly bent at the elbow but always moving straight back. The easiest way to do this is to keep the wrists flat, and to hold the poles loosely. Force your weight forward by pulling back.

Throughout, keep the poles stationary and the axis of rotation in the shoulder. Take the movement to full extension and then take it a bit further by releasing all but the thumb and the forefinger of the hand. It may take some time to get the hang of this. Once you do, however, it is quite simple.

Cross-country skiers like to use slow wheels, which duplicate the feel of their sport more closely. They also are fond of long, hilly courses.

ICE SPEED SKATING

In-line skates are playing an equally impressive role for speed skaters on the ice. Both sports use the same muscles. The in-line skates actually produce a more intense workout, because they do not coast as easily.

As a result, in-line skating has become integral to the dry-land training program of the United States Speed Skating Team. They have found it especially useful in making the transition early in the season from running and cycling to on-ice training. It also is better at teaching turning technique than any other dry land method.

The United States Speed Skating Team uses the five-wheel skate, which allows them to get into a low skate position and hold it for long periods. In addition, the wheels remove most of the vibration and the low-cut boot gives about the same support as the boots used on ice.

Speed skaters say that perhaps the greatest benefit of in-line skating is that after a cold winter cooped up in a rink going around and around in circles, they feel rejuvenated by training outside while the scenery flies past. Training doesn't seem like training at all.

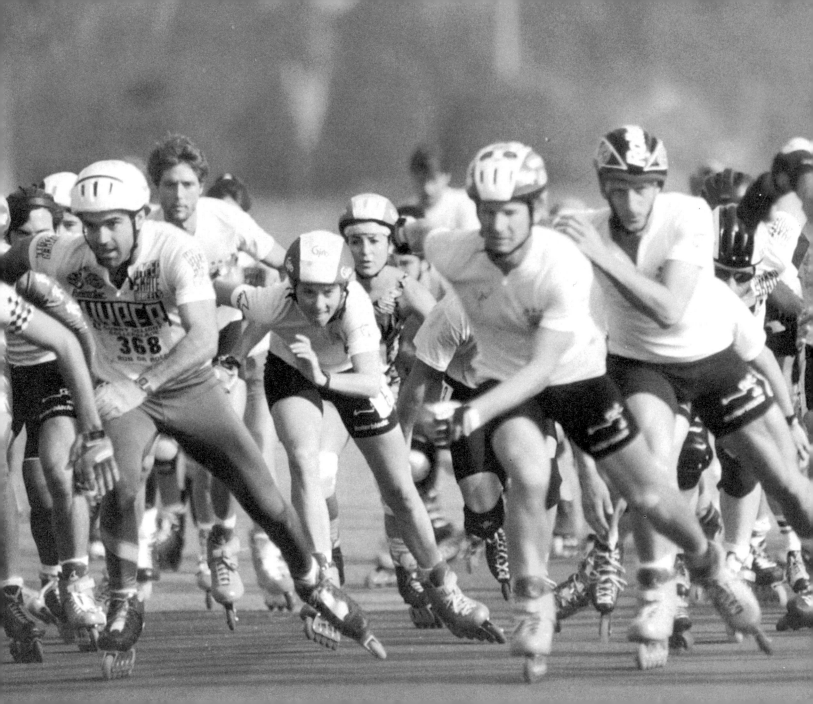

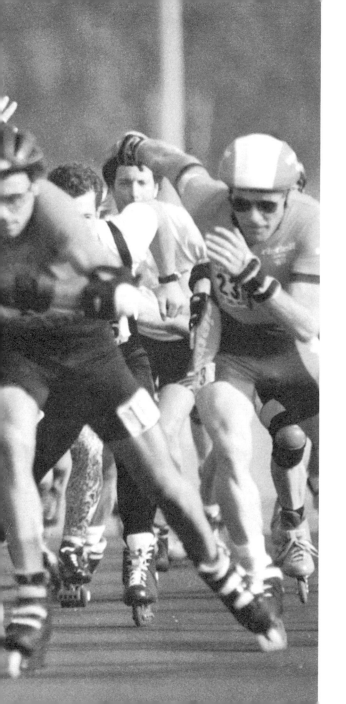

RACING

Racing is a lot like the old joke, "If you have to ask how much it costs, you can't afford it." The demanding training takes hours, and on race day you will push your physical and mental limits. But a race offers competition and speed. And to a real racer, that is reward enough.

So like the shopper who has to ask, people who have to be convinced of the inherent thrill of speed probably will remain unmoved by the appeal of the race. If the fast lane appeals to you in any way, though, you too will sooner or later end up on the race course. If you do, go out there well prepared. When it comes to racing, those who go the fastest clearly have the most fun.

Speed skating has been one of the first areas of in-line skating to generate an organized slate of events and a governing structure. At this stage of the sport's development, most organized races are 10K races sanctioned by RISA, the Rollerblade In-Line Skate Association ™. There are also shorter sprints (200 to 500 meters) and longer races, from 50 to 100 kilometers, in various parts of the country. And increasingly there are experimental offerings, such as skate-and-archery biathlons (you read that right) and relay races.

Some of the races, such as Georgia's Athens to Atlanta race, began on conventional skates, well before the proliferation of in-line skates. As in-lines proved themselves faster than conventional skates, however, all the top competitors made the switch. By 1989, outdoor speed skating belonged to the in-line skate.

BEGINNING

Because short and long races require different training techniques, the first step is deciding what kind of race you want to enter. Make a realistic decision based on your ability and your schedule. If, for example, you are a strong sprinter and are too busy to train for more than an hour a day, a 10K, which average skaters complete respectably in less than twenty-five minutes, is a better goal than a 50K. If your endurance is better than your speed, you may prefer longer distances, which reward endurance rather than quick bursts of energy and strength.

Next you have to learn racing strategy, which the best racers use as much as simple speed. Although a race looks like skaters out for themselves (and is just that near the finish line), most skaters spend most of the race with an ally or two. They use a technique called drafting, which, as you will see, gives a skater a chance to feed off the other racers' energy and skill.

THE RACER'S SKATE

Before you get to the actual race, however, you will spend weeks or, even better, months preparing for it. Make the most of your training by making your skates as fast as they can be.

Start by taking a good look at the skate's wheels and bearings. Speed skates need the highest-grade bearings the wearer can afford. But even the top bearings come packed in a heavy grease, which extends the life of the bearings but reduces the amount of speed they can generate. A few people think this helps you train because it makes you skate harder. The heavily greased bearings are, however, a real disadvantage during a race. Since most serious skaters like to simulate race conditions during their training, they take matters into their hands immediately.

They usually buy bearings with removable caps. Then they repack them by opening the cap and soaking the bearings in naphtha (a solvent) or kerosene for a few hours or even overnight. After cleaning and drying the bearings, they relubricate them with a few drops of a finer-grade oil. While not difficult, the process is dirty and time consuming.

If there is no time or if the bearings are permanently sealed, skaters can still improve their chances by soaking the bearings in a solvent for several hours or overnight. Some of the solvent will sink through the seams and remove some of the heavier grease. Complete cleaning by lubricating the seams with a white lithium or silicon-based lubricant. Enough oil will seep through to make a difference.

Even the best bearings can't salvage bad wheels, so speed skaters also spend a lot of time thinking about their wheels. Unlike conventional skates, which are fastest with the hardest wheels, in-line skates are fastest with softer wheels having durometers between seventy-five and seventy-eight millimeters. The reason is the narrowness of the in-line wheel. The harder the wheel, the more it holds its shape, so on a hard wheel you are skating on a thin, sharp edge. A softer wheel, however, slightly flattens under pressure, so it grabs more road surface. This traction can make your stroke faster and more powerful.

There is also little argument over the superiority of five wheels over four. Surprisingly, the advantage may be caused by the longer frame rather than the extra wheel. The extra length results in a longer stride, which is faster and more stable (particularly downhill). To get in racing shape, then, get the longest row of wheels suitable to your height and strength.

(Remember, however, that, while great for racing and hills, these five-wheel and long-blade models are liabilities for artistic, trick and recreational skating. Invest in them only after you are sure this is the type of skating you want to do.)

Although the boot is low cut (sacrificing ankle support for weight), it should fit the same as a regular skate— snug but comfortable. If the heel slides up and down, the boot is too big. If the toes are cramped even when you are upright or are jammed into the boot when your weight is forward, it is too small.

FOOT CARE

If you have a properly fitted boot, you can make it through a 10K training and race without giving your feet much thought. As the distances of the race and training increase, however, you may need more aggressive preventive measures. Athletic socks made of polypropylene may be more protective than regular cotton socks. Because the skate liners have edges, though, even special socks may not prevent blisters or hot spots.

When you do blister, reduce your discomfort as well as the risk of infection by covering the spot with a product such as moleskin or Second Skin. If you use moleskin, create a "doughnut" to keep a space between the blister and the skate. First fold the moleskin in half and cut out a semicircle slightly larger than half of the blister. Then unfold the moleskin. If you have cut correctly, there will be a hole in the center of the moleskin that is big enough to fit over the blister. Now the skate can move without directly rubbing on the blister. And you can remove the moleskin without ripping the already sensitive skin on or around the blister.

Since blisters tend to recur, experienced skaters tape problem areas preventively, especially when they are skating long distances. If the skin is unbroken, use the moleskin without the doughnut; a foam rubber makeup pad, which provides inexpensive but effective cushioning; standard athletic tape; or specialty products such as Second Skin or DuoDERM®.

RACING SAFELY

Racers should wear full protective gear and, if training for long distance, carry a water bottle. Remember that high-speed skating in a pack increases that possibility of a fall.

The water bottle is essential because you can lose from one to four liters of water an hour during race conditions. Your body can function only if this is replaced. Rather than run the risk of dehydration, which under severe conditions can damage the kidneys and even be fatal, replenish your water supply regularly. Rather than wait until you are bone dry, hit the bottle every fifteen minutes. And

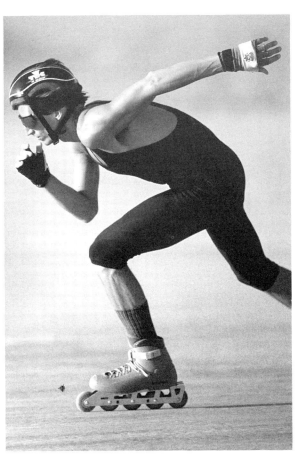

RACING STROKE

don't worry about the water causing cramps or sickness. The steady supply of water will do just the opposite, and it will help you maintain your energy level comfortably throughout the race.

Often good packs work together by continuously passing one water bottle among them.

RACING TECHNIQUES

Once you are properly outfitted, you are ready to work on techniques that will enable you to go as fast as you can for a predetermined distance. Good technique provides maximum speed at minimum effort.

One of the key elements of speed skating is the stroke itself. Take your cue from ice skaters, and concentrate on keeping the wheels in contact with the ground for as long as you can. This will not only lengthen your stroke, but will also help keep your weight forward and off the heels.

When you bring the leg back in, make sure that your knees almost touch. The most powerful part of your stroke takes place when the legs are closest to the center of the abdominal and pelvic areas. By bringing the legs in, you are far more likely to make the most of this part of the stroke.

In addition, the more the stroke goes out to the side (as opposed to behind you), the stronger it will be. To maximize its force, keep your knees pointed straight ahead and bent. It may help to picture yourself sitting in a chair with your hips back. Then concentrate on the bend in the knees, because a more pro-

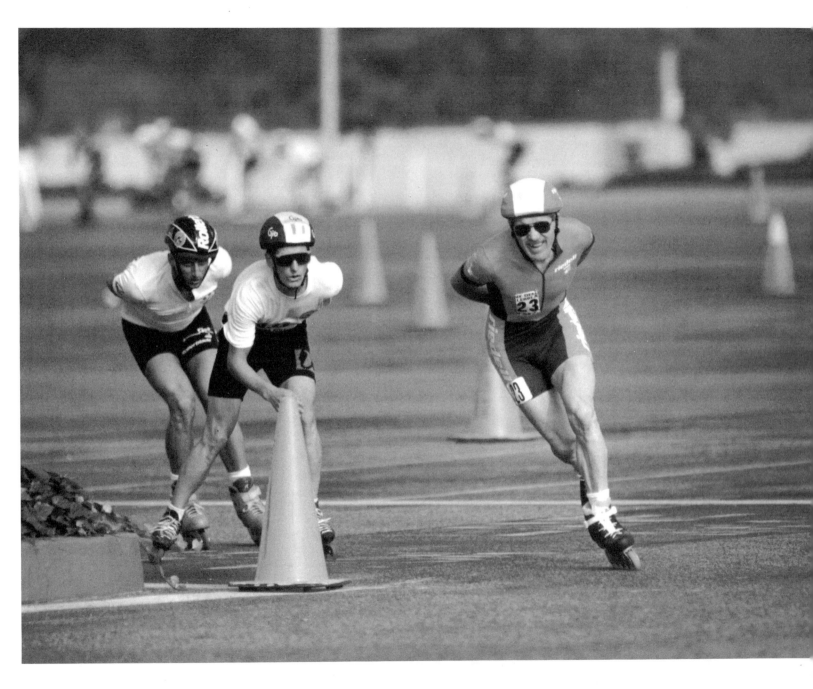

nounced bend forces you into an efficient aerodynamic tuck position. Once you get used to the tuck, further enhance it by bending forward at the waist as well.

So that you don't waste energy, keep the upper body as quiet as possible when maintaining a steady speed. For sprints or uphill climbs, gain momentum by pumping the arms in a straight line forward and backward. To hold your form, imagine that there is a rope in front of each hand and that you have to pull straight back on each to pull yourself along.

At other times, conserve energy by skating with one or two hands behind you. While this forces you into a tuck, at first it will throw off your balance. Get used to the position by practicing with one hand behind you. Then add the other. Once you are comfortable, skate in this position at a greater speed for a longer distance.

It would be great if the tuck prevented a sore back, but unfortunately it doesn't. While good training and strengthening and flexibility exercises can protect the back from serious injuries, a sore back is an occupational hazard of strenuous skating. Although rarely severe or debilitating, it does affect most long-distance or speed skaters periodically, especially as they get older. RISA urges racers with sore backs to use common sense before returning to racing.

DRAFTING

Few skills are as helpful to the racer as drafting. Technically speaking, drafting is skating inside the low-pressure area created by a skater moving directly in front of you. In the air pocket of the other skater's wake, there is less air resistance to slow you down. You thus can go faster with less effort.

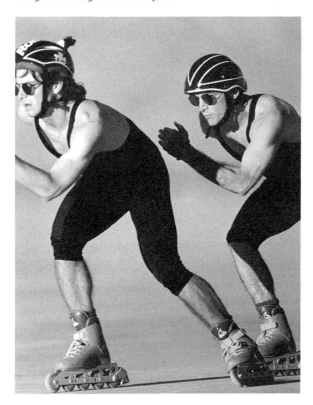

DRAFTING
The skaters are the proper distance apart, and their arm swings and skating strides are in synch.

If you trade off the lead, drafting improves your speed without compromising the cardiovascular workout. But you don't want to try to draft until you can skate well and control your balance regardless of the road condition.

Because you are skating so close to another person, you must be careful not to fall. If you are in the front, help the person behind you—who can't see a thing—by pointing out obstacles, holes in the road and turns. If you are behind, develop a feel for how close you have to get to pick up wind without endangering everyone.

Drafting is not just an important training tool, but also a critical part of race strategy. At least for the first three-quarters of the race, most of the top racers skate in a pack and conserve energy by drafting off each other. Because of the importance of drafting, the top racers tend to form teams, which have helped them win most of the races in all divisions.

Drafting works for everybody only if all the racers do their share. If you are out in front for what you feel is an inordinate amount of time and are compromising your ability to finish strongly, slow down and force someone to pass you.

But don't get left behind, particularly in short races like the 10K, where losing the pack is equivalent to losing the race. Even 100 meters are significant in a short race. To remain competitive until the final sprint, you have to stay with the pack up until the moment someone breaks away.

QUICK STARTS

In a 10K, people start by running off the start line. So that you don't trip or trip anyone else, take as much space as you can, even if it means keeping your arms outstretched.

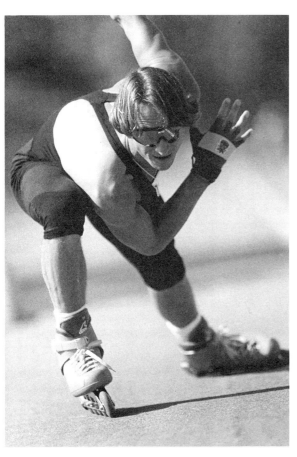

STARTING STANCE

The start is less important in the longer races, which have rolling starts with a pace car. The cars drive in front of the pack at a variable speed, giving everyone room to warm up without adding any extra mileage to an already challenging distance.

For a 10K, most elite racers warm up by slowly skating about five miles. Then they throw in a few sprints and stretches. The more highly trained you are, the longer it takes to warm up.

PACING

To complete the race successfully, you have to develop a feel for pacing. This may take some practice. At least in your first races, start out slowly. Take it reasonably easy in the first half. Then, if you feel good, turn it up.

Get an idea of your capabilities by doing half the distance of the race at full speed in a simulated race workout. The rule of thumb is that you can maintain this speed for twice the distance under real race conditions.

TRAINING FOR THE 10K

Before you start training, first build a good general fitness base by skating at moderate intensity for forty-five to sixty minutes four to six times a week. When you can do this without problems, begin training for the race.

Because the 10K is relatively short, being able to complete the race is not usually an issue. Finishing competitively is. Your performance is a result of a combination of factors, including genetics, experience and how you are feeling that day. To peak, allow yourself three months of training if you can.

Anything shorter may not prepare your muscles and cardiopulmonary system (especially for the longer races). More prolonged training, on the other hand, may make you stale.

If you have the three months, divide the training period into three parts. The first, which lasts for two weeks, helps you adjust to the increased intensity of the workout. The second, which takes from six to eight weeks, includes intensive interval training. The final segment, for the last two weeks of training, tapers off the intensity of the workouts and conserves your energy for the day of the performance.

For the first two weeks, you will be using a Scandinavian training technique called Speedplay or Fartlek training. In this game, originally developed to give runners a break from the tedium of their daily workouts, one runner led the pack at a strong pace for a short distance, then slowed the pace to allow everyone to moderately recover. He or she then passed the lead to another runner, who ran at a different speed for a different distance.

The technique of variable speeds and distances has since been adopted by many different sports. In cycling, it is called pace line; in cross-country running, it is called chasing the rabbit. Whatever the name, the principle—and the technique's effectiveness—remain the same: intense periods of exercise at about 85 percent of the maximal heart rate (see chart in Getting Physical chapter) for distances of between one-quarter to one mile with recovery periods of milder movement that last until you feel refreshed.

Speedplay improves aerobic power, but is hard on the body.

During these two weeks, you should alternate Speedplay with three workouts that cover long distances at moderate intensity. Ideally you'll want to skate for forty-five to sixty minutes at 65 to 70 percent of your maximal heart rate. Resist the urge to train longer at this point. On your off day or when you are tired, substitute an upper-body workout such as swimming or rowing or a weight workout like the one in the Getting Physical chapter. Probably best of all, take the day off and allow the body to recover.

By the third week, upgrade the Speedplay workouts to interval training. Although similar in principle, interval training is more demanding because the period of exertion is carefully controlled and at least twice as long as the recovery period.

Because the intervals are so intense, you want to work up to them gradually by beginning with about eight relatively long periods of work (three minutes) and recovery (one minute). Increase the number of periods and decrease the time spent on each so that by the seventh week of training, you are doing ten to twelve three-minute intervals with forty-five-second recovery periods, two-minute intervals with thirty-second rest periods or one-minute intervals with fifteen-second rest periods. The intervals, moreover, should be at least 80 percent of your maximal heart rate.

Because interval workouts are so taxing, give yourself time to recover between them. To ensure that recovery, do no more than two interval workouts a week. Alternate them with two long, slow distance-skating workouts and, ideally, two long, slow distance workouts in other sports. Although some people like to run or swim for cross training, most competitive skaters cycle since the sport works compatible groups of leg muscles.

Depending upon your motivation and how you are feeling,

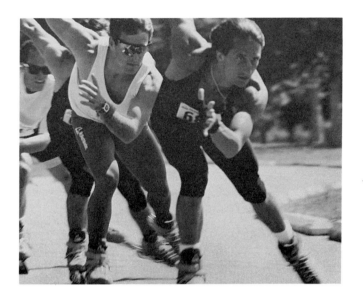

you may want to skate or bike for a long, slow distance on the fourth day of the week, or integrate a technique called repeats to help you refine your racing technique. In repeats, the skater covers short distances—usually several hundred meters to a mile—at a race pace, then skates slowly until fully recovered. Depending upon the level of training and the distance skated, the process is repeated eight to twenty times. To prevent boredom, some skaters alternate between a mile, a half-mile and a quarter mile. Others do just quarter miles. The breakdown doesn't matter because you are not trying to improve times, but instead to sharpen your technique and improve your muscular coordination. Beginners might start with four 200-meter sprints and four quarter miles, and then add four half-mile segments when they are ready. More experienced skaters can begin with four half-miles, four quarter-miles and ten 200-meter sprints.

There is ample evidence of the benefits of taking the seventh day off. It will hasten your recovery and keep you fresh mentally. If you can't stand the thought of enforced inactivity, take a walk or a slow bike ride around the neighborhood. Above all, relax. It will pay off in the end.

DAY ONE: long, slow distance skate (forty-five to sixty minutes at 65 to 75 percent of your maximal heart rate)

DAY TWO: thirty minutes of easy skating, followed by intervals

DAY THREE: long, slow distance bike ride

DAY FOUR: thirty minutes of easy skating, followed by repeats

DAY FIVE: long, slow distance skate

DAY SIX: thirty minutes of easy skating, followed by intervals

DAY SEVEN: very easy bike ride, walk or complete rest

In the third phase of the training period, the last two weeks, you are no longer concerned with building cardiovascular power. Instead, use a modified repeat workout to sharpen the race pace while conserving power. Skate at a race pace for three minutes, recover for three minutes; later reduce the time to two minutes and then to one minute. Repeat this sequence eight to twenty times.

In the eleventh week, complete one interval and two repeat workouts. Alternate them with long, slow distance workouts. One and preferably two of these should be on a bike or be another form of cross training.

Spend the last week before the race with a long, slow skate; a long, slow bike ride; repeats; a long, slow skate; a long, slow bike ride; and repeats. On the day before the race, do an easy twenty-minute skate if that.

TRAINING FOR ULTRAENDURANCE RACING

If you can do a 10K in under twenty-five minutes, you should be able to work up to a 50K and even a 100K race within three to four months of rigorous, systematic training. Remember, however, that training is like a pyramid—you cannot have a peak without a solid base.

Another critical factor in your ultimate success is that you cross train, preferably with a bike. Not only does it come the closest to working the same muscle groups, but it also allows you to remain enthusiastic throughout an otherwise grueling training schedule.

Proper hydration is essential for the longer races and in training for them. You can lose between one and four liters of fluid per hour during the race. The only way to guarantee steady performance throughout training or a race is to replace this lost fluid regularly, by drinking either water or one of the special fluid-replacement sports drinks. If you choose the latter, make sure it is at least 96 percent water. Anything less sits in the stomach too long and diverts blood from the limbs to the stomach.

To be on the safe side, drink approximately one cup of water every fifteen minutes. Adjust the amount to your weight, but the time seems optimal.

To keep your interest up and your risk of injuries down, alternate hard and easy workouts six days a week. Then, on the seventh, skate or bike for an hour at a very slow speed, without breaking a sweat, to get the kinks out.

On two of the difficult days, warm up for ten minutes and then do your intervals. One day, do about a half hour of relatively short intervals of about thirty seconds of work with about thirty to forty-five seconds of recovery at a very high intensity of at least 80 percent of your maximal heart rate. At the beginning of the training, do ten, and work up to about twenty with shortened recovery times.

On the other interval day, cut the amount of intervals in half, but double the time of exertion and recovery. Complete each interval by rolling at an easy pace for about five minutes, then do three intervals at 100 percent of your effort. This not only raises your top speed, but gets you in the habit of digging deep and finishing strong in the race.

If you have access to hills, you can do the second interval work-out on them. Ideally you want to work for twenty to twenty-five seconds up the hill and recover for thirty seconds ten to twenty times. Since shorter intervals are more difficult, you want to increase the number of intervals but reduce the length of each as you get used to the demands of training.

On the third day, use a technique called motorpacing. After asking permission, get behind someone—either a better skater or a cyclist—and draft him or her so that you can maintain a steady but faster speed than you are used to for at least an hour.

To add interest and further build your speed, get used to the rhythm for fifteen to twenty minutes. Then step out from behind and skate beside the other person—being careful to give him or her enough room that you don't collide—and go at their top speed for a minute or two. Drop back into their wind pocket for four or five minutes, and step out again. During the hour, step out at least five times. While you are behind your pacer, you should be at between 75 and 85 percent of your maximal heart rate. When you are next to him or her, you should be between 85 to 90 percent.

In between these hard sessions, build endurance by skating long distances at a relatively slow pace (between 65 and 75 per-cent of your maximal heart rate). If you are training for a 50K, you can skate that distance once a week. Go slow, have fun, practice your form and then, if you can, push hard during the last half a mile or so. On the other long skate, you can limit yourself to a maximum of 60 percent of that distance, or about 30K, also at a slower pace. On the other days or on days that you are tired, bike

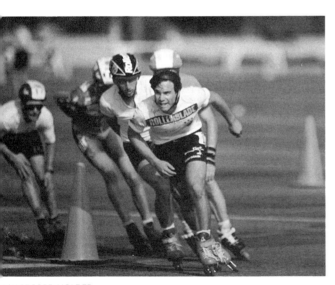

10K RECORD HOLDER

n 1990 Eddy Matzger, foreground, became the first in-line racer to break seven-teen minutes in a 10K race.

instead for an equivalent time and intensity. It is also a good idea to spend about fifteen to twenty minutes spinning on the bike after the long, slow workout days.

Before you jump on the bike, though, realize that it can be unforgiving if not set up and adjusted properly. If you are making the commitment to this type of training, don't try to get by with an ill-fitting bike. Instead, work with an experienced bike shop to keep it part of the solution rather than a potential problem.

As developed by Jonathan Seutter, world-record holder and race director for the Tour d'Malibu, the training schedule for the 50K, divided into recreational and elite levels of training, is as follows. All workouts should be preceded by a ten-minute warm-up and concluded with a ten-minute cool down.

Recreational 50K training schedule

DAY ONE: 15K pace at about 85 percent maximal heart rate

DAY TWO: long sprints or motorpace workout

DAY THREE: 25K pace at about 75 percent maximal heart rate

DAY FOUR: short sprints

DAY FIVE: 15K technique day, done at about 65 percent maximal heart rate with attention to form

DAY SIX: 50K pace at 75 to 80 percent maximal heart rate except the last five minutes, which is done at an all-out pace

DAY SEVEN: rest

Note: Use the bike to spin when you can or as a recovery tool in the pace days when you are too tired to skate.

Elite 50K training schedule

This elite training schedule is built around the principle of double workouts, spaced at least eight to ten hours apart.

DAY ONE A.M.: 30K pace
DAY ONE P.M.: bike forty-five minutes in big gears

DAY TWO A.M.: off
DAY TWO P.M.: long sprint or motorpace workout

DAY THREE A.M.: spinning workout, thirty minutes, on the bike
DAY THREE P.M.: 30K pace with fifteen minutes for technique in the middle, when you feel tired and your form becomes especially important.

DAY FOUR A.M.: off
DAY FOUR P.M.: short sprint

DAY FIVE A.M.: spinning workout, thirty minutes on the bike
DAY FIVE P.M.: twenty-minute technique-oriented skate

DAY SIX: 50K pace

DAY SEVEN: recovery

Training for the ultraendurance races of 100K and more follows the same basic training principles. These distances attract only a handful of the most serious competitors, whose incredible athletic and mental abilities enable them to add double workouts and maintain focus against incredible obstacles. Time and musculoskeletal stress, however, dictate that on the longest slow day, the skater go "only" about 70 to 80 percent of the race distance. Anything longer would interfere with recovery times and lead to burnout.

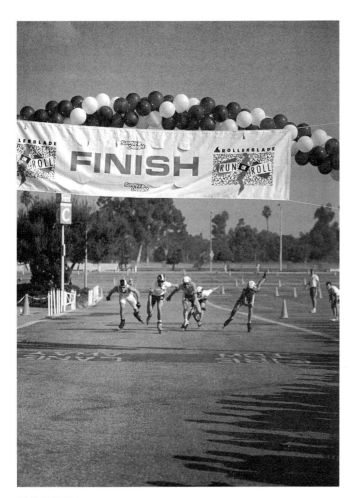

TO THE FINISH

The competition among elite in-line racers will surely increase in the future as evidenced by this sprint for the finish line at a 1990 Rollerblade race in Los Angeles.

Recreational 100K training schedule

DAY ONE: 20K pace

DAY TWO: long sprint

DAY THREE: 30K to 35K pace

DAY FOUR: short sprint or motorpace

DAY FIVE: 20K pace with five to ten minutes of technique skating in the middle

DAY SIX: 75K pace

DAY SEVEN: recovery

Elite 100K training schedule

The elite skater's training schedule uses double workouts. The bike is a training tool as opposed to a way to recover.

DAY ONE A.M.: 50K pace
DAY ONE P.M.: one-hour spin on the bike

DAY TWO A.M.: off
DAY TWO P.M.: long sprint or motorpace

DAY THREE A.M.: thirty-minute spin on the bike
DAY THREE P.M.: hills or 25K at 85 percent of your maximal heart rate

DAY FOUR A.M.: off
DAY FOUR P.M.: short sprint

DAY FIVE A.M.: thirty-minute spin on the bike

DAY FIVE P.M.: 15K slow skate with attention to technique

DAY SIX: 75K to 80K pace at 80 percent of your maximal heart rate with five two-minute sprints, each followed by a five-minute roll

DAY SEVEN: recovery

It would be a great mistake to underestimate the burnout factor inherent in this kind of training. The ability to remain emotionally flexible and motivated is as critical as the endurance and skills honed by the physical training. At the very least, have a clear idea of what you expect to accomplish by competing, and know how you can best achieve that. Work with visualization, mental imagery and other mental training tools.

Like all true competitors, filter out the thousand reasons why you can't reach your goal, and latch onto the one or two reasons why you can. When all is said and done, that is what is going to keep you going to the finish line. When it comes to racing, that's the only line worth remembering.

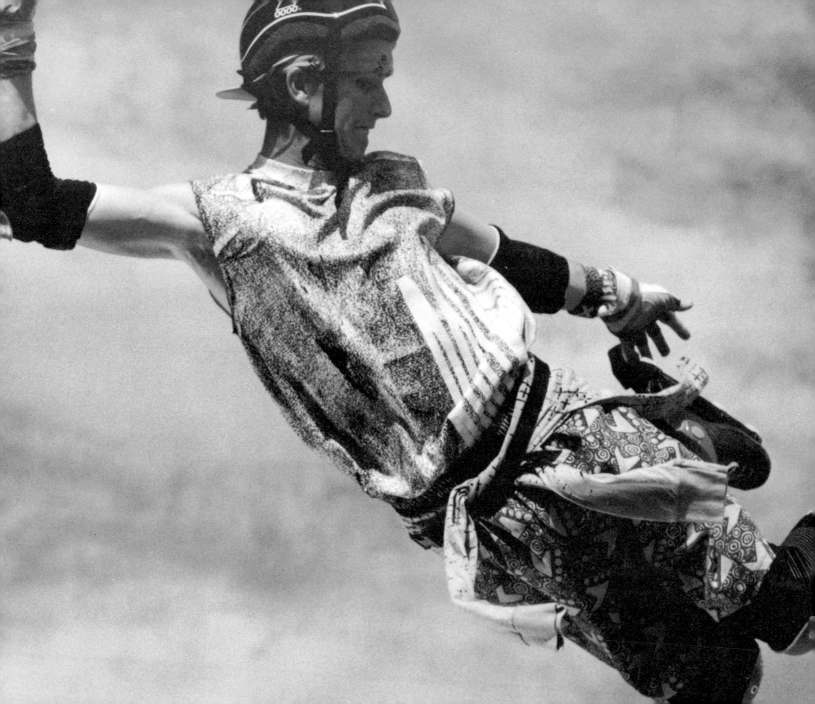

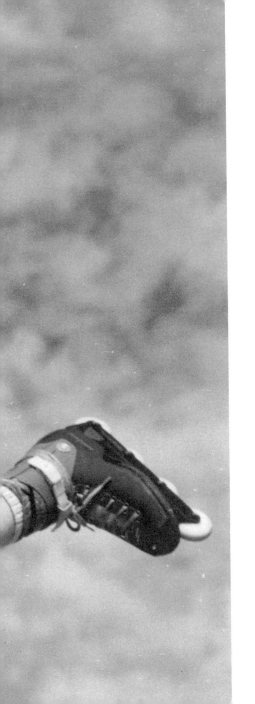

7

EXTREME AND ARTISTIC SKATING

There is not a skater anywhere who does not look at a well-executed routine, an aggressive street maneuver or an all-out stunt and deep down wish that he or she could do it, too. Be it a complicated routine, an aggressive street maneuver or an all-out stunt, the thrill of watching can only hint at the thrill of doing it.

While extreme skating is not for beginners, the faint of heart or the undisciplined, it can be done. First we'll tackle the basics of what's called with good reason "extreme skating"—stunts on the pavement, steps, walls and hills. Then we'll talk you through the glides, squats, turns and other first moves of "artistic skating," the in-line equivalent of figure skating.

Do not underestimate the difficulty or risk of these moves. Before you try them, you should be proficient at skating forward, stopping and doing crossovers. You must understand how to use the wheels as a single unit, and how to control the inside and outside edges. You must be able to skate with parallel feet and bent knees, and have enough abdominal and lower back strength to hold your form in an aerodynamic tuck. If you want to be an artistic skater, you'll have to know how to skate backward and do backward crossovers.

Needless to say, never attempt extreme or artistic skating—on pavement, a ramp or a rink—without full protective gear. It is a good idea to have a RISA-certified instructor or a spotter when attempting these moves.

EXTREME SKATING

No matter how spontaneous and effortless extreme skating may look, even the simplest tricks depend upon intense control, solid skills and practice. One of the first lessons extreme skaters learn is backing off from a maneuver or terrain they can't handle, rather than "going with the flow" and bluffing their way through a trick. This means that they always evaluate the situation before they make a move. That way there still may be a risk, but it is a calculated one.

They also become adept at breaking down each trick into manageable parts. Instead of treating a stunt as one fluid movement, they practice each element over and over, gradually stringing each one together until they can do the whole thing. After developing the confidence that comes from doing something repeatedly, they take the stunt faster, higher or more extreme.

Following is an introduction to the basic tricks of the extreme skater's trade: jumping, riding stairs or walls, jumping curbs and doing downhill, plus a few words on ramp skating.

Jumping

Start with jumping, because it is the cornerstone of all the stunts except hill riding.

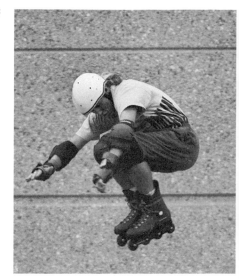

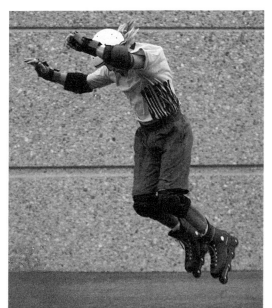

JUMPING 1

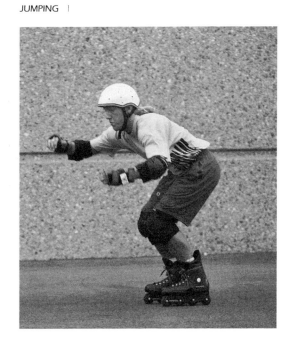

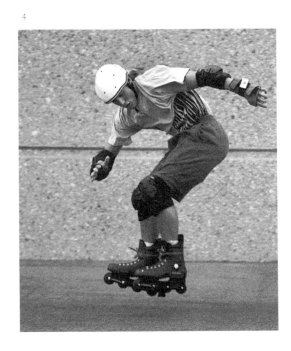

Begin by focusing on an obstacle to jump over. Although you may eventually be able to soar over taller obstacles, begin with something easier—like a crack in the sidewalk. Instead of thinking about getting your feet or skates over the object, think about clearing it with your entire body. This will help you look ahead, rather than down at your feet.

Don't be afraid to build up speed before the jump, because the momentum will make the jump easier. About five feet before the obstacle, prepare to jump. Although some people prefer to lead off with their stronger foot, you can get more lift and stability by lifting off with parallel feet. When you land, slightly scissor your feet (placing one in front of the other) and hit with your stronger foot first. This gives you a longer base to operate from when you land. As with surfing, snowboarding or skateboarding, you will instinctively know which foot works better in front for you and which one works in back. Right footers use what is called the regular foot; those favoring the left forward are called goofy footers (which some skaters consider a mark of distinction).

After the lift-off, many skaters like to grab their boots in midair. In addition to adding flair to the jump, this forces you into a tight body position, increasing your control.

Concentrate on your body, not your skates, and be ready to stride forward as soon as you hit the ground, as many street jumps end with a glide.

Once you are confident that you can clear the object, pick something slightly taller and repeat the process. Don't get impatient and overambitious, because you don't want to push yourself toward a painful injury. After all, the obstacle will be there tomorrow. You want to be, too.

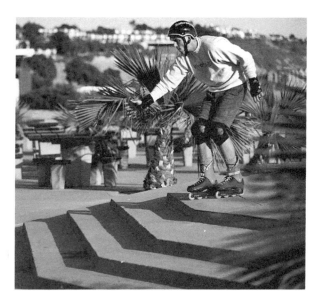

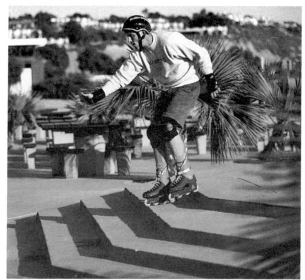

2

3

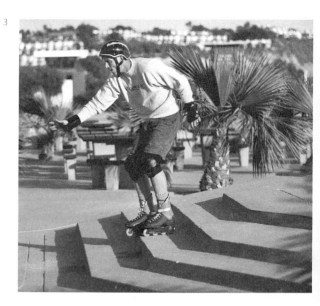

STAIR RIDING | 1

Stair riding

After learning how to jump, most street skaters turn to stair riding, or skating down a flight of stairs without losing momentum. Teach yourself to do this on stairs with a railing, holding on to it until you get used to the movement. First place your stronger foot forward, and hit the stairs with your feet about six inches apart. Keep your knees bent, your hands in front and your weight low. When you go down the stairs, the fronts of the skates may be in the air, so you cannot balance if your weight is on your toes; instead, place your weight farther back, closer to the arch of the foot and heels. Keep the front wheels straight, trail the back skate and bounce down.

Be as conservative as you were with the jumps, and pick a small flight of stairs. Once you get a feel for the movement, add one or two more steps. Don't add them too fast, because you don't want to get in over your head. In extreme skating, fear is often counterproductive.

Wall riding

Wall riding is another basic tool. Despite the name, no one has yet figured out a way to ride a wall with both skates. Instead, skaters charge the wall at an angle and make it part of the ride.

The technique is not difficult. All you need to do is get up some speed, take aim at a spot on the wall and touch the wall with the inside hand as you launch off with the leading foot. The other foot trails behind and touches but doesn't ride the wall.

Curb jumping

Curb jumping puts a twist on regular jumps. Unlike a regular jump, you do not get air by jumping. Instead, the curb gives the air to

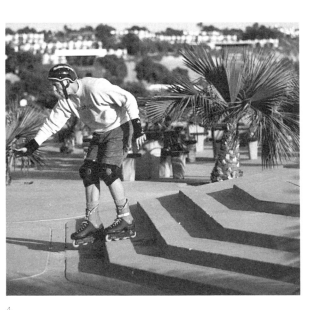

4

103

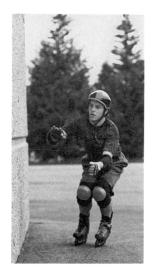

WALL RIDING

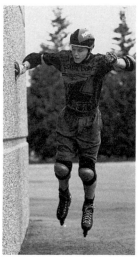

2

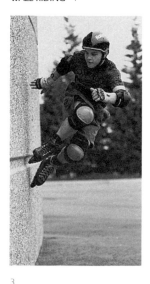

3

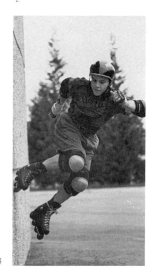

4

you. That may sound like New Age mumbo jumbo, but it's an important distinction. Although the starting and landing positions are the same as in a normal jump, the thrill of curbs is their ability to give you a boost. Merely find the top of the curb and effortlessly let it launch you.

Hill riding

Extreme skaters need to know how to navigate up and down hills. Once you have the basic skating skills, going up a hill is more a question of power than anything else. People think they have to be far forward and keep a long stride to get up hills. But it is actually easier to take short, tight strokes, so that you don't burn out. Keep your weight over your ankles, but try not to bend from the waist since that will tire you out. Instead, stay relatively upright with your back straight and your weight on the balls of your feet rather than the toes or the heels.

Going down is a different story. Short of wearing an air bag, you have no choice but to learn control. Even though "running a hill" is one of skating's greatest rushes, falling on one is its biggest nightmare. So never charge a hill without being sure you can handle it first. Don't even think about skating down hills until you are adept at stopping while going full speed.

Then, to get down, you should know how to skate with your weight forward and on the balls of your feet. Stay in the tuck position, and slightly scissor your feet for stability. Your arms should remain immobile, which will enhance your stability further, and your head should be down with your eyes forward.

Although it may seem safer to stand up straight, that is a sure

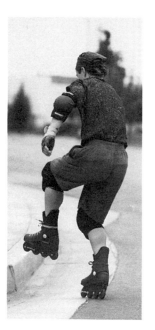

CURB JUMPING 1

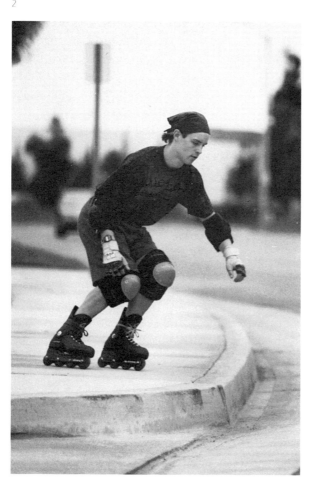

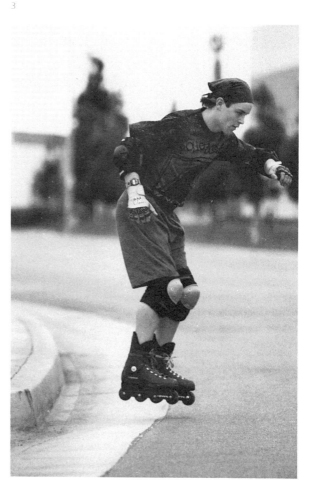

way to fall because your weight is pushed back to your heels. This not only makes the turns more difficult to control, but increases the likelihood of the skate going out from under you. Since a hill is the last place you want to fall, this would be a big mistake.

It would be equally foolish to go down a hill without first making sure there are no stop signs or opportunities for unobserved cross traffic. Even if there aren't, make sure you are visible at all times.

Don't think that you can be cavalier about this and, if you get into trouble, that you can cut your speed by traversing down the hill. This may be an effective option for the experienced skier or skater, but it can be a difficult maneuver that throws anyone else off balance. If you do traverse, use quick, simple, committed turns, which are easier to control than wider ones. Keep your weight on the downhill or outside foot. Do a fast turn, then glide perpendicular to the fall line or even slightly uphill. And remember that this is a next-to-last resort.

As far as braking goes, it too is a matter of sooner rather than later. If you are not sure of your ability to make it down, begin braking well before you hit full speed and certainly before you lose control. Once you get scared or out of control, braking is not as effective and can actually throw you further off balance.

When faced with a potentially dangerous situation, take off your skates and walk down the hill. You can always put your skates back on, skate up a bit, race down the part you feel comfortable with and gradually piece together your ability to make it down the entire hill.

Finally, although you never want to fall on a hill, it is a good

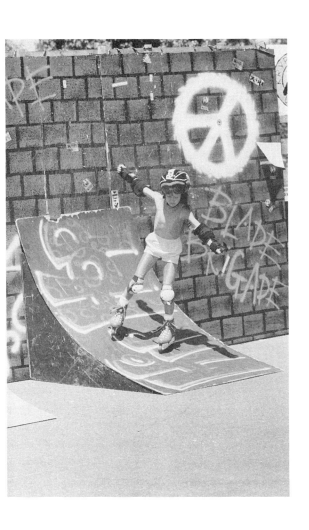

idea to learn how to fall properly. As with any other skating skill, practice it first on the grass in street shoes or socks so you get used to the move. As you begin to fall, tuck your shoulder and your head in, and fall to one side. Then roll or tumble over and slap your hand on the ground. The wrist guard will protect you, and the slap will absorb the shock and help stop the fall.

Ramps

Lastly, there are ramps. Although most ramp skating gets quite technical and difficult, here are a few basics.

The first kind of ramp you will probably deal with is a launch ramp. To propel yourself off it, approach it with enough speed to match how high you want to go. Keeping your weight square in the center and your arms in front, sink into the road with a deep knee bend. Glide for at least ten feet before you hit the ramp, go into a tuck and give yourself a little spring right before you hit the top.

A big problem in the launch ramps is the fear factor, which causes you to keep your weight on your heels and fight any forward momentum. To help you keep your weight on the balls of your feet, you can bring your arms up in a bent position, shoulder width apart, which should help keep your weight forward.

Land in a slight scissor position with the knees slightly bent to absorb the shock of a landing. Then sink down further to absorb more of it.

The other two kinds of ramps are the half-pipe, which has two peaks and a valley between, and the quarter-pipe, which has only a peak and one valley.

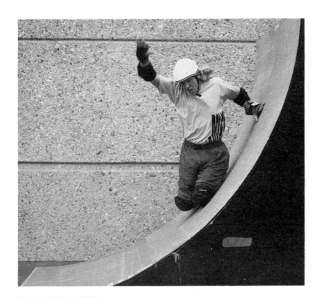

SLIDING TO SAFETY

The knee pads are designed to let you slide safely down the ramp. If you find yourself in this position, point your knees down to the ground, which will increase the likelihood that you land in the transition area. You want to do this because a fall in that area has less shock than one on a flat area.

The first skill to learn on a quarter- or half-pipe involves gyrating, or pumping the ramp. Begin with a good stride so you can work your way into the transition (the part of the ramp that goes from horizontal to vertical). The key here is to loosen, rather than tighten, the legs so that there is no added pressure that will cut your speed. You ultimately want to feel your weight move from your legs to your upper body, and the best way to do that is to keep any pressure off your feet and keep a bend and flex in the knees.

Then, as you get to the top and are about to stop, turn your arms in the direction you feel most comfortable in. Pull with one

180-DEGREE TURN ON A QUARTER-PIPE

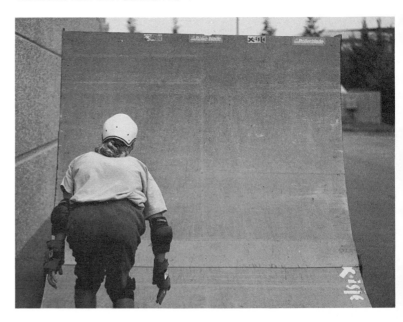

hand down and the other up, and commit to a 180-degree turn. You can do this simply by scissoring your arms and slightly pivoting your feet. The one thing you do not have to do is push off the ramp with your skates, because that will only eject you.

As you head to the bottom of the half-pipe, extend your leg out again, keep a flex in the knees and get speed for the next transition. This obviously is not an option in the quarter-pipe.

Because of the risk involved, the best way to learn these skills, as well as the more advanced ones, is by going to Camp Rollerblade® or by learning from a RISA-certified instructor.

2

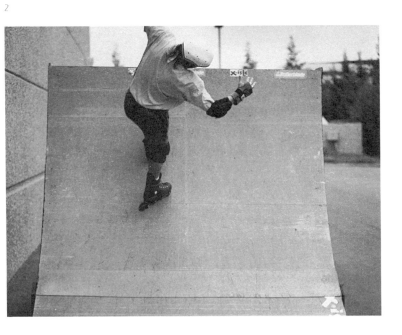

3

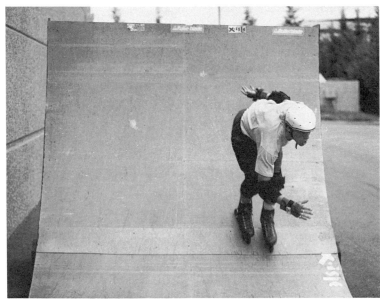

TOUCHING THE TOP

This is a way to add flair to the ride.

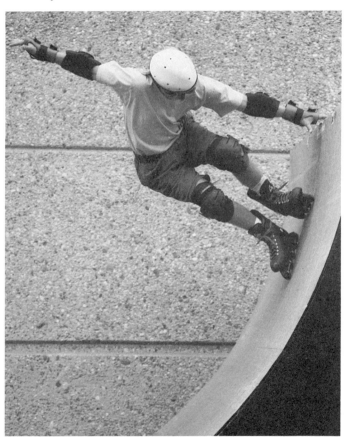

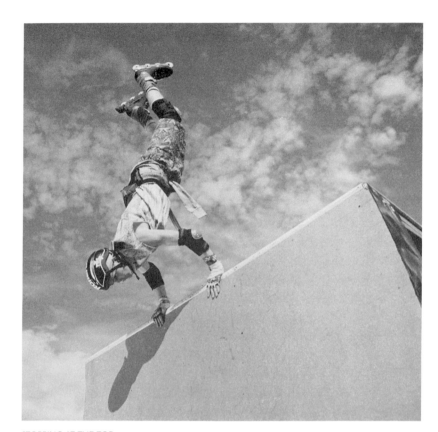

STOPPING AT THE TOP

This move is optional and purely a matter of style

ARTISTIC SKATING

Although ramp skating is often intricately choreographed, chore-ography is even more closely associated with artistic skating. Artistic skating is based on figure skating on ice, and it looks very similar. The only notable exception, in fact, is the one-foot spin, which can-not physically be performed on in-line skates, yet.

Because choreographed artistic skating demands considerable technical expertise, it is best taught by a coach. If no in-line skating coach is available, work with a dance instructor or ice-skating coach.

Although the following instructions will not replace lessons, they will give you a sound foundation in the basic moves. Since the skills build upon each other, you should learn them in the order they appear.

The glide along

To glide, first go on to the toe of the back foot. Then lift the front toe, so that you can move onto the front heel. At first, feel free to practice while holding onto something, just so you can get used to being up on the wheels. Once this feels comfortable, you can add the movement.

1

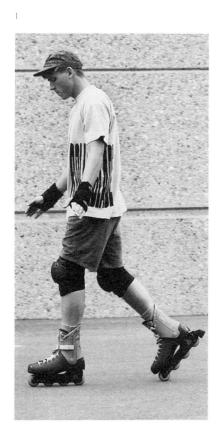

2

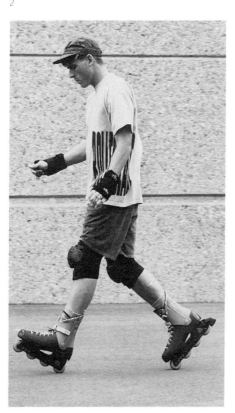

3

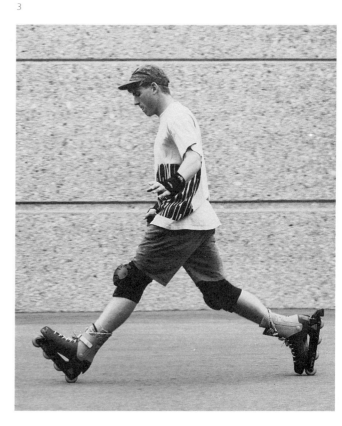

Low squats on one foot

With the same foot in front, get on the toe of the back foot. Keeping your weight over your knees, squat so that you are sitting on your heels. Remain on the toe of the back skate and glide with the other full row of wheels. Balance equally on both legs. Keep your hands in front of you or, for added stability, on the front knee.

Although this movement may sound difficult, it is easier than it looks. Just squat straight down and don't drop the knee all the way down to the ground; if you do, you'll come to a sudden stop.

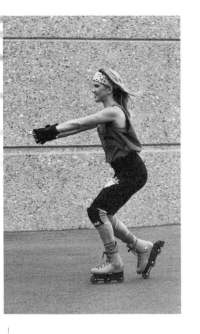

1

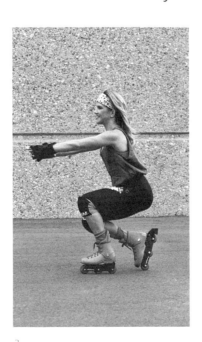

2

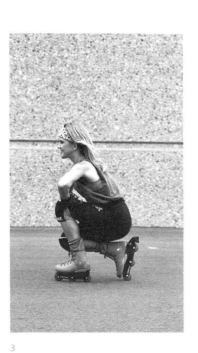

3

Up on both toes

This movement uses the same principle as the heel/toe balance in the glide along. Build up a moderate amount of speed and put one foot slightly behind the other. Go up on the toe of the back foot first. Then, with your weight evenly distributed and over the knees, bend the other knee and lift up on the other heel.

So that you don't lose your balance, make sure the skates do not line up side by side. Once you can easily balance, practice keeping your momentum up by swiveling the hips and toes. At first, though, you'll have enough to do just holding your balance for the duration of the glide.

1

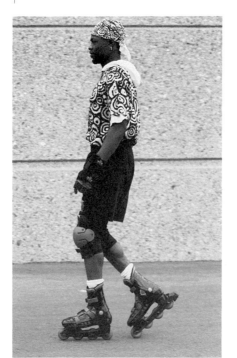

2

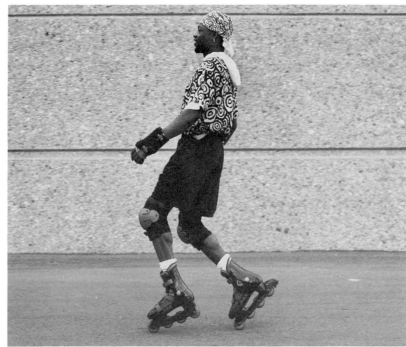

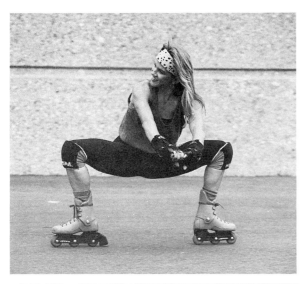

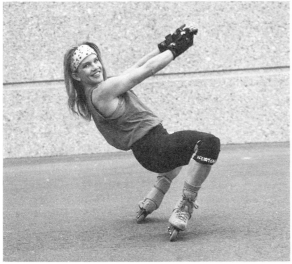

The spread-eagle squat

The spread-eagle squat with both feet turned out is another maneuver that looks more difficult than it is. This is particularly true if you know how to control your inside and outside edges. In addition to being an impressive display, the spread-eagle squat can also be a flashy, fast way to switch from forward to backward skating.

Since most people find it easier to turn to the left (counterclockwise) when going from front to back, the instructions describe this directional swing. If you want to turn right instead, reverse the foot positions.

Begin by stepping forward on the right inside edge. Turn the left toe out and bring the left foot down on the outside edge so both toes are out and under the shoulders. Push with the left foot and glide into a curve on the inside edges. Next, pick up and place the right foot. Keeping your weight on both legs, squat down with bent knees. Then stay on top of the row of wheels so that you can glide. The further you squat, the more you will warm up the inner thighs and reduce the risk of inner thigh and groin injuries.

To help develop a feel for this movement, find a skating partner. Hold hands facing each other. Turn the toes of both feet out, push with the left foot and glide on your inside edges. You will then automatically go into a counterclockwise turn that gets you used to the turned-out stance. Later, after you become advanced, work on leaning back, which is called cantilevering.

CANTILEVERING

115

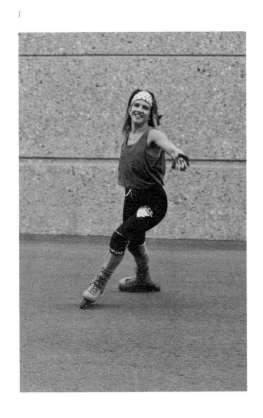

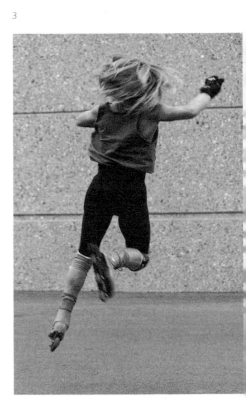

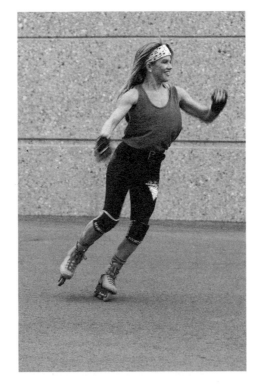

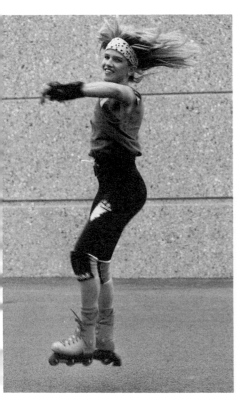

The 360-degree jump

As with the spread-eagle squat, the instructions describe a jump to the left, because most people find it easier to start in that direction.

Skate forward at a moderate speed, so you have enough momentum to complete the turn. With bent knees, take off from both feet—on the left outside and right inside edges. As you go up, swing and pull your arms in. Slightly curve your body to turn and at the same time slightly lift your feet up. Do one complete turn and come down in the same position you started in.

Advanced skaters add another 360-degree turn afterward, or do 180-degree turns, which ironically are more difficult than the 360s.

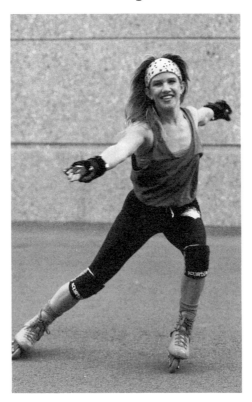

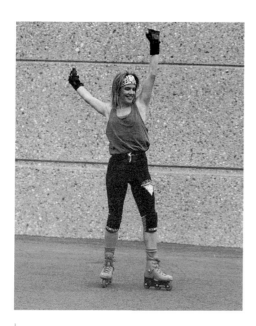

Cartwheels

If you can do cartwheels without skates, doing them on skates shouldn't be too difficult. If you can't, first learn how to do them in shoes. Once they become easy, find a spot of level grass or a carpet. Learn to do cartwheels on skates here first, so you can get used to the skates' added height and weight.

To go into the cartwheel, stand with your feet in a wide T-position. While standing still, decide where to plant your hands. Lift the arms slightly, and place the hands straight down as you kick your legs over. Don't think about the wheels; treat them as a single, solid, immobile row. Set your right foot down, and get back to the T-position as soon as possible so the wheels don't roll. This should bring you to a stop and allow you to keep your balance.

When this becomes easy, go to the border where the grass meets the concrete. Let a friend spot you from behind, and practice launching from the grass and landing on the pavement. Then change directions and start from the pavement and end up on the grass. After you are comfortable with both, move completely onto the pavement. Then, when you get comfortable, try doing consecutive cartwheels, cartwheels that begin while you are moving and, when you are really good, one-handed cartwheels.

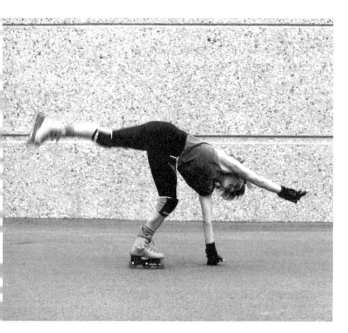

2

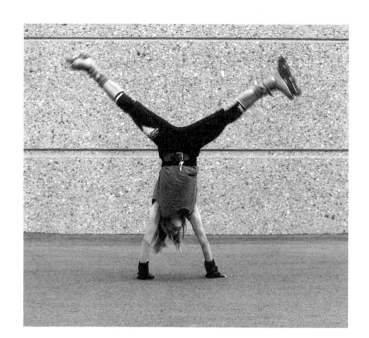

3

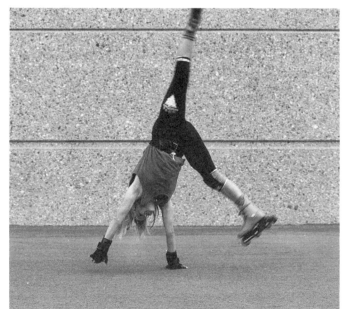

4

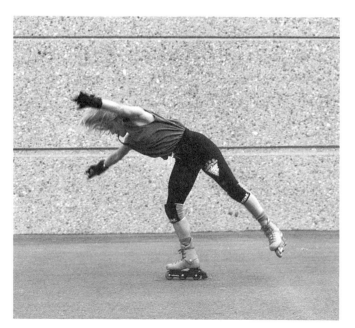

5

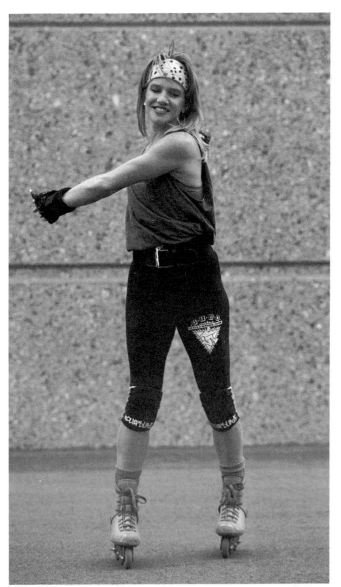

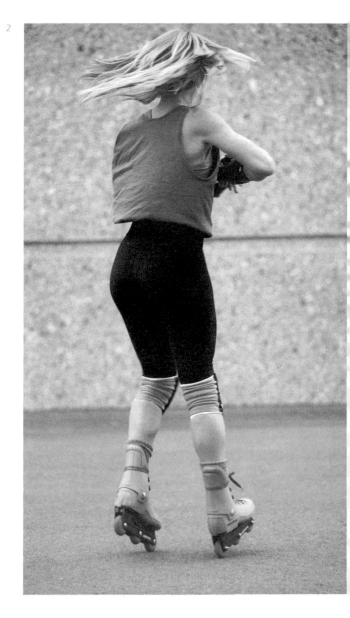

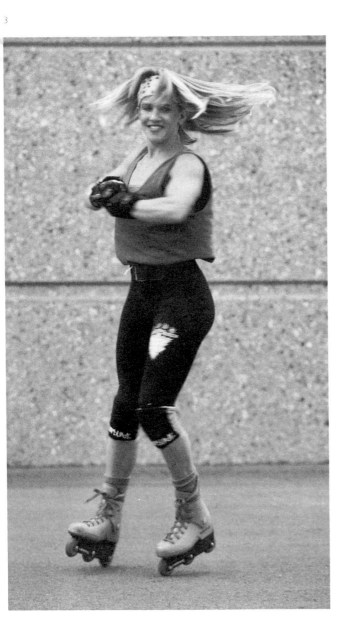

The spin

Undoubtedly most impressive of this grab bag of tricks is the spin. Since most skaters turn to the left here as well, the instructions will remain slanted in that direction.

First find a completely flat, smooth surface. Anything less will complicate your life tremendously. Remove the heel brake, because it will interfere with the spin (therefore, skaters doing a spin must know the T-stop or power stop). Stand still with your feet slightly apart under your shoulders. Bend your knees slightly. Keep your arms out from your sides. Twist your shoulders a little to the right to begin.

All that follows next has to happen at once. Twist your arms and shoulders to the left. With your momentum to the left, pull the arms directly into the chest. Slightly lift the right toe so that you are on the right heel. Go onto the left toe, and stay with the spin for as long as you can. As you practice, the spins will get longer. If you pull your feet toward each other, they'll also get faster.

Spirals

Work up moderate speed going forward in a straight line on a flat surface. With the knees bent, find the foot you can best balance on and shift your weight there. Keep your arms stretched out to the side, turn the opposite hip out and extend the foot of that leg out at a 45-degree angle. Practice your balance at this angle. When you are comfortable with this, bring the leg into the full arabesque position by hinging the hips slightly forward so that the leg and chest move parallel to the ground. Once the leg is extended, slightly straighten but don't lock the standing knee. Keep your arms to the side to prevent a tilt.

1

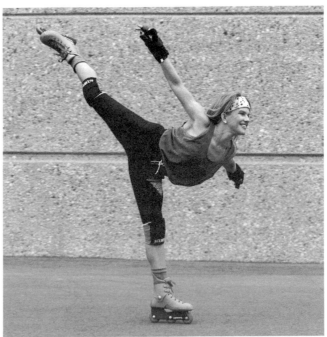

2

As artistic and stunt skating becomes more established, expect increased interest in organized competition. Present competitions feature three areas: half-pipes; streetstyle, which includes quarter-pipes, launch ramps, wall rides and other jumps; and "Hip Hop," which features individuals, pairs or groups with choreographed routines. In all three competitions, participants will have a set amount of time to display their skills, and will be judged on a scale of one to ten by a panel of officials. For more information on these artistic and stunt competitions, call 1-800-255-RISA.

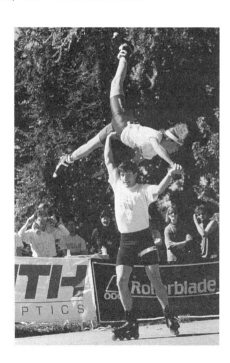

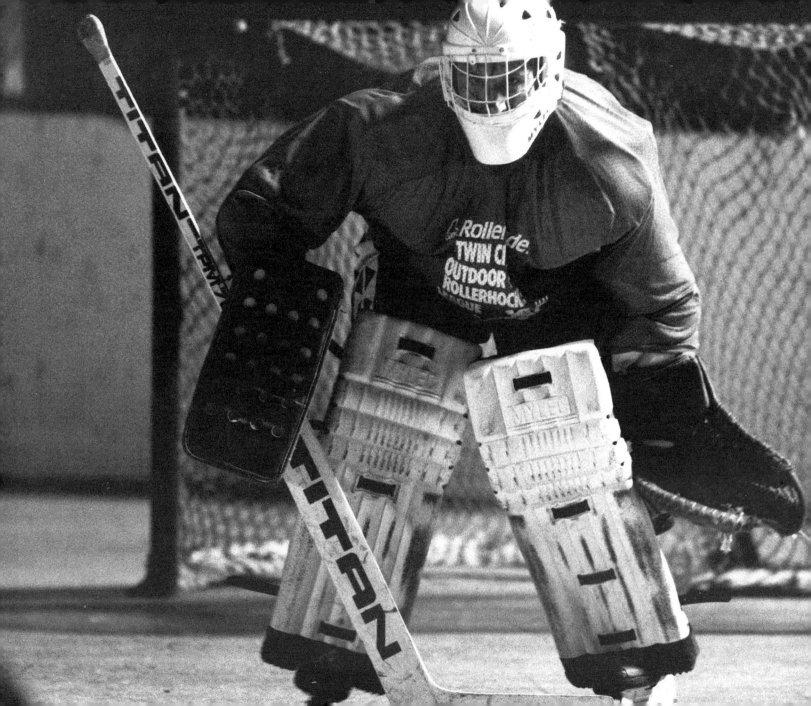

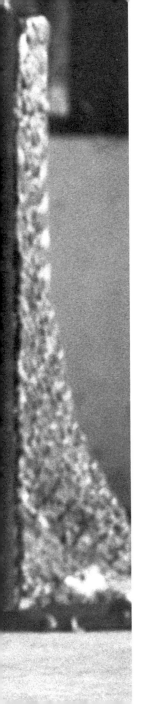

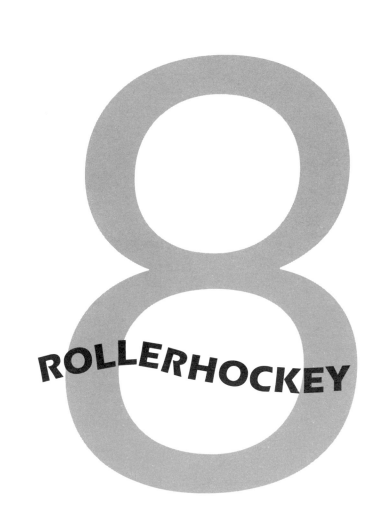

ROLLERHOCKEY

With rollerhockey leagues opening up all across the country, in-line skating has come full circle. The skates were first developed by ice-hockey enthusiasts searching for an off-season cross-training tool. Now rollerhockey has become a sport of its own, drawing skaters with no previous hockey experience as well as converts from the ice.

The number of rollerhockey players is growing rapidly. And why not, since this fast-paced, rugged sport offers all the thrills of ice hockey, without the need for an ice rink. And within the in-line skating world, it is probably the best place to experience the special joys of being on a team—the team pride, the camaraderie and the shared victory.

For information on leagues in your areas, call 1-800-255-RISA.

THE BASICS

Like ice hockey, rollerhockey is played with a weighted puck and wooden hockey sticks. But unlike ice hockey, which can only be played outdoors in cold climates and indoors at rinks, it can also

BOX STRATEGY (goalie not included)

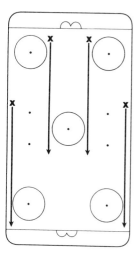

DIAMOND STRATEGY (goalie not included)

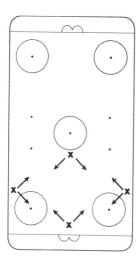

work on driveways, basketball courts, tennis courts, roller rinks and out-of-commission ice arenas.

It is a more wide-open game. Rather than six players, roller-hockey teams have five, including one goaltender, two defensemen and two forwards. Checking (contact) is not allowed, so the players have more room and opportunity to move the puck up the rink. Also, there are no offsides calls; this means skaters can move up the entire rink (usually 180 by 85 feet) in an effort to find an opening to score goals without worrying where the rest of their team members are.

The lack of an offsides rule results in more end-to-end excitement, more breakaways and fewer stops in the action. To accommodate the added physical demands and faster pace, rollerhockey games are limited to two fifteen-minute halves, rather than the three periods of ice hockey.

There is one overriding similarity between ice hockey and rollerhockey: The object of both games is to put the puck into the net more often than your opponent does.

PLAYING THE BOX

There are two schools of thought on how best to score goals. The first, which is favored by experienced rollerhockey players, is the "box" or "diamond" strategy. The team forms a square like the one in the upper diagram, and moves up the rink as a unit, passing the puck to each other. This continues until they move close to the opponent's goal. They then take turns breaking for the net. They try to get open so they can receive a pass and from there, shoot for a goal.

To add diversity to the attack, the team rotates its square and forms a diamond similar to the one pictured in the lower diagram. The theory remains the same, but the positions change.

Like basketball's four-corner offense, this tried-and-true strategy can be an effective way to protect a lead or score goals through short, crisp, relatively safe passes. Yet it is conservative, because the whole team works as a unit with the defensemen always in the back so they can help the goalie if necessary.

BREAKING OUT

The second option, the breakout strategy (pictured in the diagram) is less conservative, because it permits team players to skate around the rink haphazardly, looking for ways to get free, accept long passes and score goals. Like the box, play begins with a defenseman starting out from one side of his net. Depending upon his position, he then will pass the puck either to the other defenseman on the other side of the ice, or to his forward along the boards or to the forward who started at center ice and is skating toward the other side of the boards. If none of the others are in place or if he sees the right opening, he can also maneuver around his opponents and carry the puck up the rink himself.

If there is time once the players get the puck near their opponent's goal, they usually revert to the box or diamond. If not, their only alternative is to shoot.

The breakout strategy encourages more aggressive maneuvering, longer passes and more frequent scoring opportunities. But because it is less controlled, it also gives the other team more

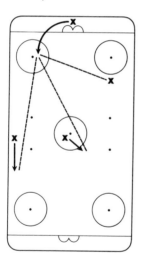

BREAKOUT STRATEGY (goalie not included)

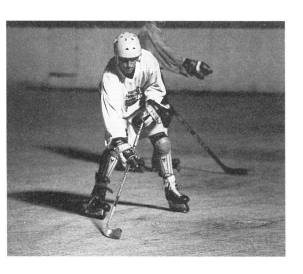

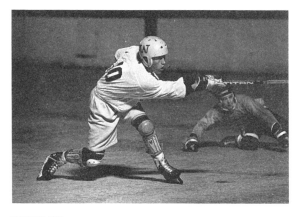

WRIST SHOT

The hands are positioned correctly, and the follow through is high.

chances to score—especially when a team gets caught up in the excitement and forgets to play defense. Because the skaters are moving randomly, it is much easier for an opponent to get open and to be ready for his own breakaway to the other end of the rink.

Because the strategies in rollerhockey are basically limited to the box and the breakout, most successful teams spend their time practicing their basic skills rather than developing elaborate game plans.

Successful teams also assign each player to the most appropriate position. The question of who plays where is critical. All hockey players need to know how to stop and start quickly and have to be accomplished sprinters. Each position also requires other more specialized skills.

THE FORWARD

Because the forwards must do the most sprinting—to break free from the opposing defensemen, accept passes or score goals—they should be the most physically fit members of the team. This is even more important in rollerhockey than in ice hockey, because coasting is more difficult on the heavier in-line skates. The amount of skating leads most teams to carry at least two sets of forwards.

In addition to being able to skate long distances, forwards must have "soft hands," or be able to easily receive passes. They also need a quick, accurate wrist shot, which will let them capitalize on openings provided by the goalie, and will help them compensate for the dimensions of the net (3 1/2 by 5 feet compared to the 4-by-6-foot ice-hockey net). The corners are most difficult for a goal-

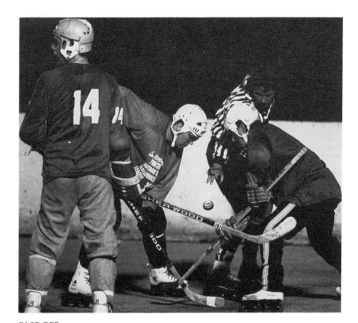
FACE-OFF

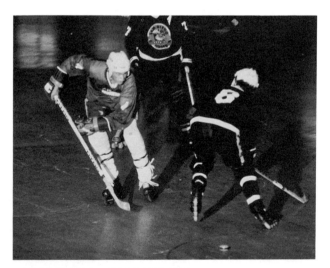
DEFENSEMAN RIDING OUT AN OPPONENT

tender to protect; so forwards should practice shooting wrist shots to all four corners of the net.

Forwards should also learn how to control face-offs, which occur at the start of a period, after a goal or after any stop of play. As in ice hockey, a referee drops the puck between two players, who then try to backhand it to one of their teammates.

THE DEFENSEMAN

Because checking (contact) is illegal in rollerhockey, such defense skills as riding the player out (see photograph) and stealing the puck are important.

Although the defenseman, like the goaltender, has to be careful not to drop to his knees to try and stop a shot, he must also be committed when confronting an opponent with a puck. When defending an opponent, a defenseman is often skating backward, which is slower than skating forward. The defenseman should therefore try to steal the puck or force a pass before the opponent builds up a head of steam. This makes a breakaway and goal less likely.

Since there are only four team members moving the puck, if only the two forwards can put the puck into the net, the team will have limited scoring opportunities. The best defensemen can move the puck up the rink and also demonstrate offensive skills such as passing, stickhandling, shooting accurately and maneuvering around an opponent. Also, since most of the defensemen's shots will come from the top of the box or diamond, a defenseman must develop an accurate, low, long-distance slapshot either to score or to set up a forward, who can either tip the puck in or tap in a rebound.

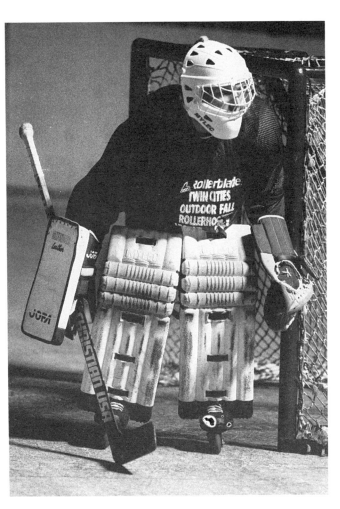

GOALTENDER IN THE PREFERRED STANDING-UP POSITION

However, no matter how intense the play gets, the defenseman must remember that his primary role is defense. He may be in the attack zone trying to score a goal, but he always has to keep an eye on the other team. Because there is no offsides rule, one of his opponents can slip away, get down the rink and be open for a long pass. A good defenseman not only stays back whenever the other defenseman is shooting or close to the opponent's goal, but learns to prevent breakaways by always being aware of the opponent's position.

THE GOALTENDER

The goaltender needs the quickest reaction time on the team. He also has to be able to follow the action so he can keep his eye on the puck. Goaltenders are the only players that have to learn how to catch the puck in their gloved hand.

The goaltender must learn not to skate out too far or to drop to his knees to stop a shot. If he does either and misses, he has over-committed himself to the play and is less likely to recover. This is a serious mistake because a rollerhockey puck, which is lighter than an ice-hockey puck, is likely to curve, drop or rise and therefore has to be closely followed by the goaltender if he is to prevent a score.

The best way to do that is to remain standing and continually cut down the opponent's shooting angles. The only time the goalie should drop to his knees is in a last-ditch attempt to smother the puck.

Because the puck used in rollerhockey is quite lively, a rebound gives any opponent who is hovering around the net a terrific opportunity to score. If the goaltender is on his knees, he will be unable to block it and prevent the goal.

THE POWER STOP

When watching rollerhockey, the first skill people usually notice is the "power stop." Unlike the heel or T-stop, the power stop is accomplished by sharply placing the front foot sideways at a sharp angle. The friction caused by the wheels rubbing against the pavement stops the player faster than the other two forms of stopping. This advanced technique should be learned from an accomplished rollerhockey player. Novice players who try to teach themselves run the risk of turning an ankle.

1

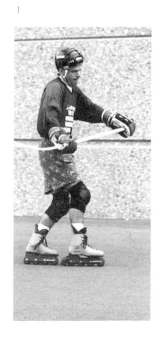

2

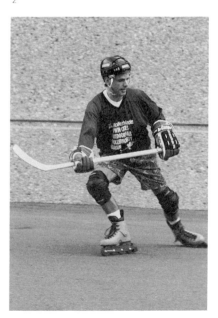

3

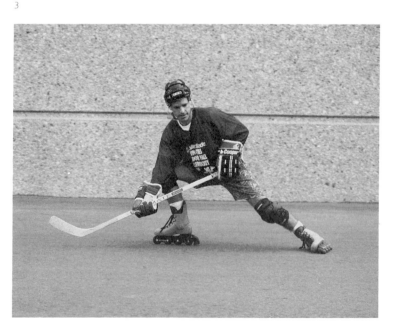

Because the game is fast and demanding, you need the right equipment. Don't try to get by with ice-hockey equipment, which will be too heavy. Instead use the lightweight equipment designed especially for rollerhockey.

Begin with a good, lightweight helmet that has a face shield, a pair of strong work or Bandy gloves and elbow pads. Since checking is not allowed, you won't need shoulder pads or padded pants. To avoid embarrassing rear-end abrasions, though, you'll probably want to wear sweatpants or short-style ice-hockey pants without the pads. Padded knee and shin pads are mandatory; probably the most effective of these are ice hockey's referee shin guards, which include knee pads.Men are required to wear a protective cup.

Stick length is a matter of personal preference. Most forwards like shorter sticks, which are easier to handle. Defensemen prefer longer sticks, which help them steal the puck.

Since the goaltender is directly in the line of fire, he should wear a lightweight mask, a chest protector, a protective cup, a lightweight blocker (which lets him hold a goaltender's stick), a lightweight glove to catch incoming pucks and lightweight leg pads.

Regardless of your position, you'll want to rocker your skates. By placing the front and back wheels higher than the center ones, you give the row of wheels a U-shaped appearance that sharpens your turns. Although other types of skaters also rocker their skates, it is most important for rollerhockey players.

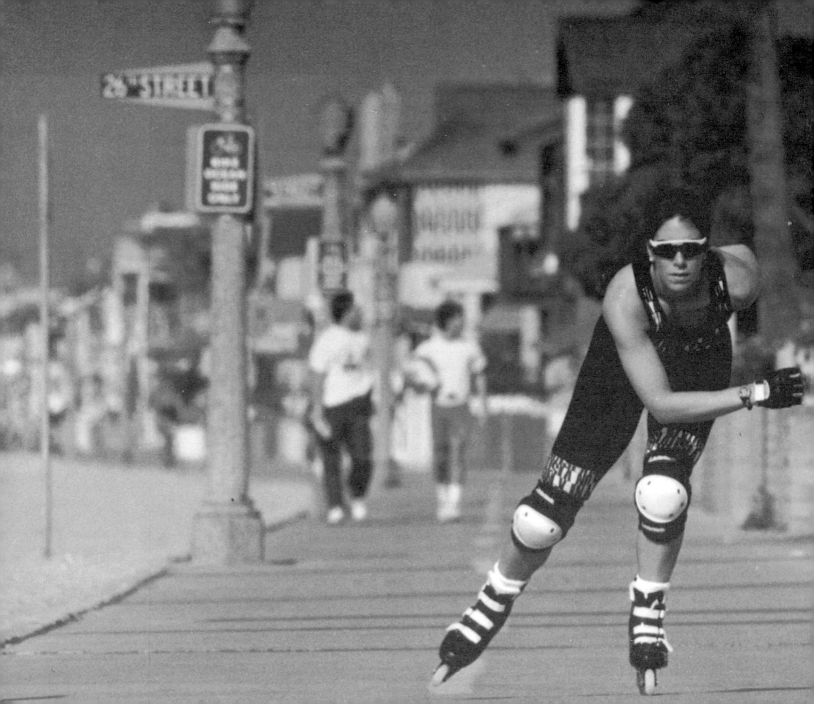

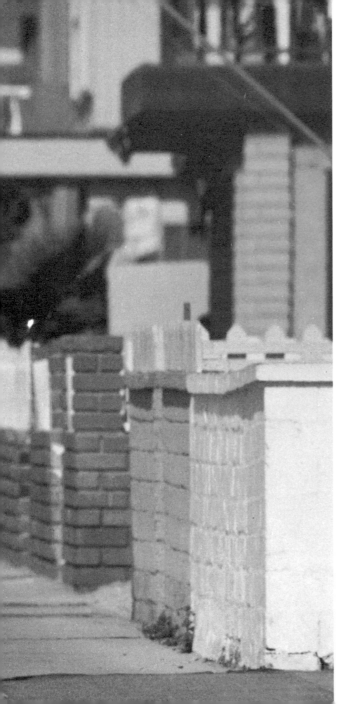

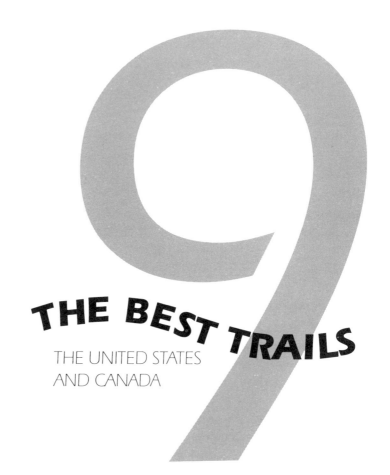

9

THE BEST TRAILS

THE UNITED STATES
AND CANADA

What makes a skating trail great? Scenery? A smooth, broad skating surface? Freedom from pedestrians and cars? Terrain? Or is it just easy parking, good lighting and easy access to refreshments?

The answer, of course, depends upon your own needs. But in any case, save perhaps the last, you can find a growing number of great paths for skating. Although the following list of trails is by no means complete, it highlights many of the country's best existing trails. These trails are generally wider than ordinary bike paths, which allows for the skater's wide stride, and/or are closed to pedestrians.

With this list, you'll be able to take along your skates when you travel for business or pleasure, knowing you won't miss out on the area's top trails.

Before long, the network of skating trails should be truly national. In the future, skaters will be able to enter marked trails assured of a safe, pleasant workout. Working toward the establishment of a recognized national system, the Rollerblade In-Line Skate Association and the Minneapolis architectural firm of Dahlgren, Shardlow and Uban have created guidelines for in-line skating trails. These guidelines cover everything from trail width to gradients to fall areas and dividers. If you want to work with your local city and country parks and recreation departments to establish safe, enjoyable skating paths, you can obtain these detailed guidelines by calling 1-800-255-RISA.

Some of the trails described below are "rail trails," trails built on abandoned railroad beds. For a complete list of these nationwide, call the Rails to Trails Conservancy at 202-797-5400.

Whether you're jamming on a California boardwalk, enjoying a Rocky Mountain high or cruising around a Minneapolis lake, on these trails you will have not only a great time, but also good company. To keep the good times rolling, always follow the Rollerblade Rules of the Road.

THE ROLLERBLADE® RULES OF THE ROAD

1. Stay alert and be courteous at all times.

2. Control your speed.

3. Skate on the right side of paths, trails and sidewalks

4. Overtake other pedestrians, cyclists and skaters on the left. Use extra caution and announce your intentions by saying, "Passing on your left." Pass only when it is safe, and when you have enough room for both of you to be at the full extension position of your stroke.

5. Be aware of changes in trail conditions due to traffic, weather conditions and hazards such as water, potholes or storm debris. When in doubt, slow down. Do not skate on wet or oily surfaces.

6. Obey all traffic regulations. When on skates you have the same obligations as a moving vehicle.

7. Stay out of areas with heavy automobile traffic.

8. Always yield for pedestrians.

9. Wear safety equipment: wrist guards, knee and elbow pads and a helmet.

10. Before using any trail, achieve a basic skating level, including the ability to turn, control speed, brake on downhills and recognize and avoid skating obstacles.

UNITED STATES TRAILS

ARIZONA

Arizona's climate makes it a year-round haven for in-line skaters. One of the state's best trails is located in south Phoenix outside South Mountain Park, which is the world's largest municipal park. Parking can be found at the intersection of Baseline Road and 40th Street. The trail runs four miles before coming to Circle K Park, where there are restroom facilities. From there skaters can take another loop around the park or continue on the trail another 2.6 miles to 7th Avenue. The trail is very smooth and flat, which makes it suitable for beginners, but is also great for race training because it has several miles of uninterrupted straightaways.

Other top trails include the Greenbelt Trail in South and North Scottsdale, Lake Mary Road in Flagstaff, Catalina State Park in Tucson, Desert Breeze Park in Ahwatukee and the downtown skating tour of Mesa, which starts at the Mesa Southwest Museum and passes thirty-eight outdoor plaques describing Mesa's history.

PHOENIX, ARIZONA

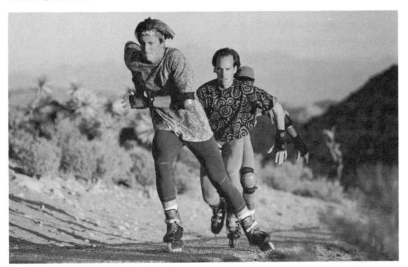

CALIFORNIA

There are probably more in-line skaters in Southern California than anywhere in the world, because of both the climate and the access to some of the world's most dramatic coastal bike paths. Both tourists and locals train or just coast the long boardwalks along Mission Beach in San Diego, Newport Beach and Huntington Beach in Orange County, Long Beach and the thirty-mile stretch of path between Redondo Beach and Santa Monica (which passes through Venice).

There is also an excellent inland path in, of all places, the Valley. Exit Ventura Boulevard from the Sepulveda Freeway in Encino, a northwest suburb of Los Angeles. Go west on Ventura Boulevard to White Oak Avenue to Victory Boulevard. Go east on Victory to Balboa Boulevard. Turn right on Balboa and park at either the Sepulveda Dam Recreation Area lot or the dirt lot across Balboa near the archery range.

The five-mile loop begins on the bike path at the intersection of Victory and Balboa boulevards. Go west along the bike path to White Oak Avenue. Turn left on White Oak and left again on Oxnard. Stay on Oxnard until you get to Balboa Boulevard. Then turn right. If you need to use the restroom or want to eat or drink something, head for the Balboa Sports Center. Otherwise, stay on Balboa to Burbank Boulevard. At the intersection of Balboa and Woodley, turn left and follow the bike path under the traffic. Veer left onto Woodley until you hit Victory. Turn left and skate back to your start.

Although less glamorous than the beach trails, this is one of the best beginner trails in Southern California because it is smooth and flat and because it separates the pedestrians from the people on wheels. It is also well-lighted so night skating is a possibility. It is the site of a weekly free in-line skating clinic, which takes place at the intersection of Burbank and Balboa boulevards. To make a reservation for the clinic, call 714-827-7655.

Perhaps with the exception of Central Park in New York, San Francisco's Golden Gate Park is the most diverse in-line skating park in the country. As might be expected in this most eccentric of cities, skaters can be found jamming to their own kind of music or bombing down the notorious San Francisco hills to the oceanfront. The park is filled with skaters on Sundays, when motor vehicles are prohibited.

Bay area skaters also like the Embar-cadero or Sawyer Camp Trail, a six-mile trail overlooking Crystal Springs Reservoir.

COLORADO

The diversity of Colorado's in-line trails matches the majesty of the surroundings. Denver offers Washington Park, the site of the local Rollerblade Run or Roll Race. Nearby Boulder offers the eleven-mile Boulder Bike Path.

Advanced skaters will enjoy the long Canyon Recreation Trail, set in the middle of some of Colorado's most popular ski resorts. Start in Keystone or Breckenridge. From Keystone, the trail winds 6.5 miles to Dillon and another 5 miles to Frisco. From Breckenridge, the trip is 10 miles to Frisco. From Frisco, skaters can travel 5.5 miles to Copper Mountain Resort. There they can travel 7 miles to the top of Vail Pass and 14 miles down to the town of Vail. Remember, this trail is for advanced skaters only.

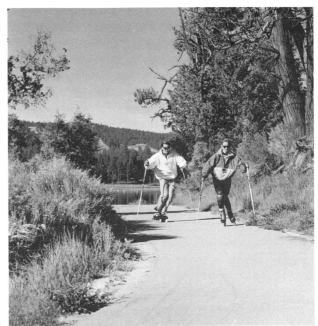

IN THE ROCKIES

DISTRICT OF COLUMBIA

Washington, D.C., has some of the longest and most scenic trails in the United States. For a trail featuring the national monuments and other points of interest, start at the intersection of 24th Street and Virginia Avenue. Skate east and circle the Lincoln Memorial, the White House and the Washington Monument. Continue east toward the Capitol and catch a glimpse of the Supreme Court. Then skate along the National Mall past the Smithsonian Institution, skate south around the Jefferson Memorial and the Tidal Basin, past the Lincoln Memorial again and head back to where you started from.

To get farther out of the city, skate the Washington and Old Dominion Railroad Trail, which runs a challenging forty-five miles from Arlington to Purcellville, Virginia. The path offers a variety of asphalt surfaces and has mile markers throughout. There are numerous towns along the way that offer restrooms and food.

Other trails of note include the three-mile loop around the East Potomac Golf Course and the five-mile Rock Creek Parkway, both of which are closed to motor traffic on Sundays; the ten-mile trail on the Mount Vernon Trail that follows the George Washington Parkway and the Potomac River; and Freedom Plaza near the White House, where an in-line skating club meets on weekends.

FLORIDA

With its wide sidewalks along the Atlantic Ocean, the east coast of Florida is probably a break-out area for in-line skating. But people living on the gulf side have their share of skating areas, too—the Boca Grande Path near Fort Myers, for example. It is located on Gasparilla Island. Get to the island through Charlotte County to enjoy this path, which cuts a primarily straight 6.5-mile trail through the center of the island.

Farther up the Gulf Coast is the Tallahassee–St. Marks Historic Railroad Trail, which is a former railroad bed now covered with asphalt. The sixteen-mile trail attracts many skaters, most of whom are students at Florida State University.

Not to be outdone, FSU's rival University of Florida, located in Gainesville, has an extensive system of bike paths that are increasingly popular with the state's growing number of in-line skaters.

GEORGIA

Atlanta has a particularly rich skating history, because of its 84.5-mile road race from Athens to Atlanta each October. Atlanta's Piedmont Park is a fine skating area, suitable for both beginners and more experienced skaters interested in training.

ILLINOIS

Chicago boasts Lake Shore Drive, where in-line skaters can roll for miles along Lake Michigan. For a change of pace, intermediate skaters may want to skate up and down the ramps that extend at a 30-degree angle along much of the route.

For a rural view, try the Fox River Trail, forty-five miles west of Chicago. This thirty-two-mile path runs along the Fox River from Algonquin to Aurora, and is an eight-to-ten-foot-wide trail that runs along the river through forest preserves and city parks.

MASSACHUSETTS

Most in-line skaters in Boston like to skate along the Charles River, but Southwest Corridor Park, a five-mile, one-way trail that begins at the Westin Hotel near Copley Place and runs from the

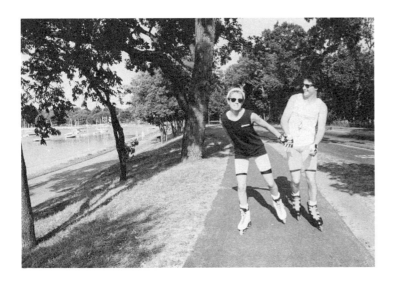

LAKE HARRIET,
MINNEAPOLIS

Back Bay to Franklin Park, is also recommended.

Skaters in this area may want to join the Great North Road Rollers for their in-line races in Burlington and Stowe, Vermont, including the annual Roll Vermont race.

MINNESOTA

Since Minnesota is Rollerblade, Inc.'s home state, it is fitting that it boasts some of the country's best skating trails. Most of the trails are located in the Twin Cities of Minneapolis and St. Paul and are part of a system linking the city

parks and lakes. The trails separate skaters and cyclists from pedestrians. Skaters frequently outnumber both other groups on the paths.

The most popular area is Minneapolis's Chain of Lakes. If you park at the Theodore Wirth Golf Clubhouse off Highway 55 and Theodore Wirth Parkway, you can follow the bike/skate trail north six miles to Webber Park or south one mile to Cedar Lake. From Cedar Lake, skaters can skate around Lake of the Isles (2.9 miles), or also add Lake Calhoun (3.4 miles) and Lake Harriet (3.2 miles). At the southeast corner of Lake Harriet, skaters can also take a

ten-mile trip along Minnehaha Falls and then add further distance with a 2.5-mile loop around Lake Nokomis. All trails are smooth and flat, and are perfect for the beginning in-line skater.

From Minnehaha Falls, skaters can use the trails along West River Road and go for 5.5 miles to Washington Avenue near the campus of the University of Minnesota. They can cross over the Mississippi River to St. Paul at Franklin Avenue or Lake Street and skate the same distance along East River Road.

There are numerous other in-line skating trails in St. Paul. The most popular starting point is the parking lot at the south end of Lake Phalen, located at the intersection of Wheelock Parkway and East Shore Drive. The trip around the lake is a level 3.1 miles. Ambitious skaters may add 5.3 miles to their skate by following Johnson Parkway to Indian Mounds Park. Another well-used path is the shorter 1.8-mile loop around Lake Como, which is near the intersection of Lexington Avenue and Midway Parkway.

Although most Minnesota skaters favor city trails like these, growing numbers who want longer, less crowded trails have discovered the 19.7-mile Cannon Valley Trail in Cannon Falls, the

12.5-mile Douglas State Trail in Rochester, the twenty-eight-mile Heartland State Trail in Park Rapids and the thirty-two-mile Willard Munger Trail in Hinckley.

NEW YORK

In New York City, the premier skating spot undoubtedly is Central Park, which prohibits motor traffic from 10 a.m. to 4 p.m. on weekdays and throughout the weekend. Skaters can take long excursions around the park, slalom through cones placed three feet apart down a hill or dance on the flats of the mall.

In upstate New York, a much more serene trail is the 6.2-mile trail at Onondaga Lake Park in Syracuse. This is a smooth, level course that has restrooms and concession stands, and is open from March to October. Parking is available at Griffin Stadium and Long Branch. The twelve-mile Colonie Niskayuna Bike Path in Albany is more challenging, because it contains some hills. It runs from the Mohawk River to Knolls Atomic Labs.

PENNSYLVANIA

There are several short in-line routes near Philadelphia, but skating is making inroads throughout the state. The five-mile loop round North Park Lake in North Park, which is located in Glenshaw, a suburb of Pittsburgh, is popular with beginning and intermediate skaters. Presque State Park near Erie is a 5.3-mile-long (one way) scenic trail, which snakes around lagoons, a nature center and Presque Isle Bay. The park, a peninsula reaching into Lake Erie, has ample parking and restroom facilities.

TEXAS

In the Lone Star State, in-line skating is still a growing sport, so the trails tend to be shorter than in other more established skating centers. The Dallas area is a particular hot spot, with many skaters flocking to the multipurpose trails in the city of Arlington. The best trail in this system, whose paths generally are less than a mile and a half, is in the River Legacy Parks, which has a 2.66-mile trail along the Trinity River.

Another good trail is in Longview, 125 miles east of Dallas. The Cargill Long Park Trail is 2.5 miles of smooth asphalt, and is excellent for beginners. The trail can be reached through Teague Park, which is close to the National Guard Armory.

WASHINGTON

In Seattle, a town with numerous skating opportunities, the most popular remain Seward Park and Green Lake. For a longer jaunt, check out the Burke Gilman Trail, which starts in Gasworks Park in Seattle and roams twenty-five miles along the Lake Washington Ship Canal to Redmond. Skaters can also skate the King County Interurban Trail, which runs sixteen miles from the town of Tuckwila (at South 180th Street) through North and South Kent to the town of Pacific.

CANADIAN TRAILS

ALBERTA

The Mill Creek Ravine Trail near down-town Edmonton may be the best in-line skating trail in Alberta. Take the 86th Street Exit from 63rd Avenue and park at the Argyll Velodrome. There are restrooms and refreshments at the Velo-drome and at Cloverdale Park at the end of the trail. The wooded, 4.5-mile trail has many small hills, so it is best suited for intermediate skaters.

ONTARIO

Toronto may be the ice-hockey capital of North America, so it has lots of cross-training skaters and rollerhockey play-ers. A favorite route is the flat, beginner, eight-mile Don Bicycle Route near Edwards Gardens. Park at Victoria Park Avenue or Don Mills Road, which both run north of Don Mills Parkway. Skaters can add four miles by skating the Sunnybrook Park System, which begins where Don Mills Road intersects the Don Mills Parkway; this beginner trail travels near the Ontario Science Center and Sunnybrook Hospital. Skaters can also add the 12.4-mile Martin Goodman Trail, which intersects the Mills Route at Cherry Street and Lakeshore Boulevard. It starts along the Eastern Beaches and travels along the shore of Lake Ontario to popular tourist areas such as Harbor Front and Ontario Place all the way to Sunnyside Park. Some parts of the Goodman Trail are more skatable than others, but the entire trail can be used by beginners. Because of the traffic on the trail, skaters looking for a long, uninterrupted workout are advised to avoid weekends and afternoons.

BRITISH COLUMBIA

Vancouver is known for great downhill ski areas, so the most popular in-line trails cater to skiers. One of the best is the Seymour Demonstration Forest Trail in North Vancouver, thirty minutes from downtown. Access the trail from the Mount Seymour Parkway off North Highway 1. Drive three miles, past Capilano College, until the road ends at a parking lot. The trail off the parking lot is a limited-access vehicle road that is open to the public on weekends and sometimes during the week. It is seven miles of good pavement. This is not a loop trail, so turn around at the mile marker of your choice. The steep hill near the six-mile mark should be attempted only by advanced in-line skaters with ski poles.

A Vancouver trail suited for skaters of all abilities is the Endowment Lands on the campus of the University of British Columbia. Follow West 16th Avenue to the parking areas at Pacific Spirit Regional Park. Skate west on the bike trails that weave through the campus. The trails are connected to acres of paved parking lots offering wide-open skating areas.

ABOUT THE AUTHORS

Neil Feineman is the publisher of *Beach Culture* magazine, the author of eight books related to fitness and health and a longtime long-distance in-line skater. He lives in Los Angeles.

Team Rollerblade® is a group of professional in-line skaters who serve as ambassadors for Rollerblade® products and the safety, fun and fitness of in-line skating. In the group are top racers, rollerhockey players and skaters who specialize in extreme or artistic skating. The members of the team have a variety of backgrounds including professional dance, ice figure skating, hockey, skiing, skateboarding, racing and acrobatics. Team Rollerblade has performed throughout the United States, Canada, Europe and Australia. Performances have included the Super Bowl, *Today*, the U.S. Olympic Festival and NBA half-time shows.